Clinical Cases
in Dermatology

Robert A. Norman • Justin Endo

Clinical Cases in Geriatric Dermatology

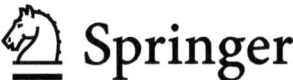 Springer

Dr. Robert A. Norman, DO
Tampa
USA

Dr. Justin Endo, M.D.
Madison
USA

ISBN 978-1-4471-4134-1   ISBN 978-1-4471-4135-8 (eBook)
DOI 10.1007/978-1-4471-4135-8
Springer London Heidelberg New York Dordrecht

Library of Congress Control Number: 2012950987

Springer is part of Springer Science+Business Media (www.springer.com)

Series Preface for Springer Clinical Case Reports Books

It is my great honor to be the series editor for the Springer Collection of Dermatology Case Reports Books. The case report format is a wonderful tradition and is particularly important in today's rapid-fire times.

Proposed Series Books will include Geriatric Dermatology, Inflammatory Disorders, Sexually Transmitted Diseases, Integrative Dermatology, Atopic Dermatitis, Dermatological Surgery, Wound Care, Malignant and Benign Neoplasms, Bullous Diseases, Hair and Nail Disorders, and other important subjects. Each book of didactic cases is of great practical help to both experienced and novice dermatologists. Although each book's primary audience is dermatologists, it can also provide guidance to internists, family physicians, and emergency room doctors.

I believe that each book in this series will greatly contribute to the education of those that carefully study and read the cases. My great hope is that the patients of every practitioner that has absorbed and applied the lessons in each of these books will benefit from these case studies.

I have worked with Grant Weston and the staff of Springer for many years and I know they produce consistently excellent books and have a wide distribution and international readership. Thanks to Grant and all the Springer people for their hard work and energy.

Thank you to all the wonderful authors for their insight, time, and determination to bring each book to fruition. Each of these books reflects the contribution that these talented authors and editors have made to add more light to the art of medicine and the care of our patients.

Dr. Rob Norman

Preface

The demographic imperative has reached the shores of dermatology. My great desire in contributing to this book is to add to the preparation that we as dermatologists and physicians need to care for our aging population in the years ahead.

After World War II we built more schools, trained more teachers, and created more playgrounds to gear up for the explosive birth rate. Not only does the post–World War II generation have more members than any other generation but will also live longer. By 2020 the aged 65 years and older will comprise a fourth of the US population, and this demographic change will be even more significant in less developed countries.

Our time has come. It is our duty to care for the aging boomers. As a specialty, we are in enormous need of increasing our skills to respond to this unprecedented demographic shift. Over the last several decades, dermatologists have enjoyed a sustained achievement in our basic scientific knowledge and proven effectiveness of clinical interventions. As dermatologists, we need to be at the top in providing specialized care and health care delivery for older adults. We must be at the forefront of prevention and treatment of skin diseases and be able to recognize the dermatologic signs of chronic systemic disease so often noted in our elderly.

The book includes chapters on autoimmune disorders, infestations, premalignant and malignant lesions and neoplasms, inflammatory disorders, drug eruptions, and cases involving hair and nails.

I am grateful to the enthusiastic medical students, Joseph Salhab & Jenny Chen, who helped perform literature searches, gather articles, and facilitate this project. I would also like to thank Ibsen Morales for administrative support. Working with a rising young star in the field of geriatric dermatology and academic medicine, Dr. Justin Endo, has been a pleasure, and my great wish is that Dr. Endo will continue to help bring the field of geriatric dermatology to center stage within the huge arena of dermatology.

Dr. Rob Norman

Contents

Part II   Infestations

Part III   Premalignant Lesions and Neoplasms

Part I
Autoimmune Disorders

Chapter 1
An Elderly Female with Blisters

An 82-year-old female presented to the office with her daughter and daughter-in-law complaining of painful blisters on the legs and arms that had occurred cyclically for the past 6 months (Fig. 1.1). She became hospitalized and bed-ridden.

Based on the case description and the photograph, what is your diagnosis?

1. Bullous drug eruption
2. Pemphigus vulgaris
3. Bullous pemphigoid
4. Epidermolysis bullosa acquisita
5. Bullous scabies

Following her hospitalization, she was moved to her daughter-in-law's home. After 1 month, the daughter-in-law noticed malodor emanating from the patient's legs, raising the possibility of superinfection. The patient also complained of pruritus and pain. She was hospitalized, the bandages were removed, and multiple tense serous blisters were noted from the mid-calf to the feet.

The patient had temporary symptom relief with oral steroids but quickly had recurrence after steroid taper was attempted three times. The patient noted discoloration, thinning and dryness of her skin.

R.A. Norman, J. Endo, *Clinical Cases in Geriatric Dermatology,* Clinical Cases in Dermatology, DOI 10.1007/978-1-4471-4135-8_1, © Springer-Verlag London 2013

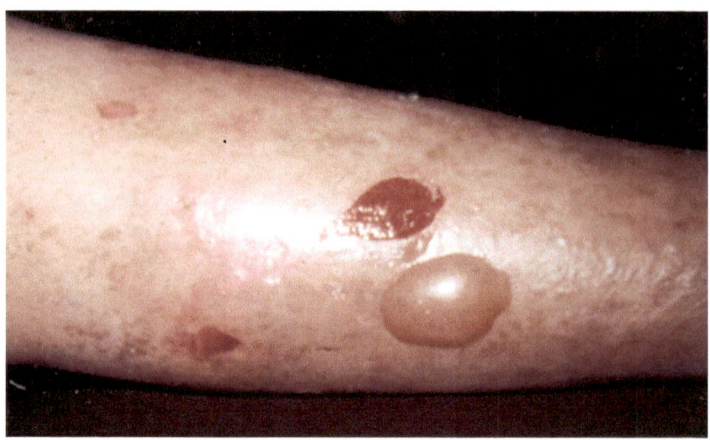

FIGURE 1.1   An 82-year-old female presented complaining of painful blisters on the legs and arms that had occurred cyclically for the past 6 months

Biopsies for direct immunofluorescent studies were obtained from perilesional skin on the right shin and right buttocks and were positive for linear junctional IgG and C3.

Diagnosis

Bullous pemphigoid

Discussion

Bullous pemphigoid, which is caused by autoantibodies that are directed against proteins at the dermal-epidermal junction, is an immunoblistering disease (Abbas et al., 2005). The autoantibodies are directed against the hemidesmosomal proteins BPAG1 and BPAG2. The blister develops at the lamina lucida of the epidermal basement membrane, hence the clinical appearance of tense blisters, which separates the lamina densa from the plasma membrane of the basal cells. This is followed by an activation of complement, as well as recruitment and activation of neutrophils and eosinophils. The blistering lesions result from the interactions with the material released from the inflammatory cells (Johnson et al., 2005).

This disease generally affects the elderly. The lesions appear as tense, fluid filled bullae. They can be pruritic and associated with erythematous or normal skin, but sometimes can have an urticarial appearance. Lesion distribution is often the inner thighs, flexor surfaces of the forearms, axillae, groin, lower legs and lower abdomen. The lower legs are often the first site of manifestation. Bullous pemphigoid has also been linked to other disorders, such as diabetes, rheumatoid arthritis, dermatomyositis, ulcerative colitis, myasthenia gravis, and thymomas (Bolognia 2008). Many cases of bullous pemphigoid enter into remission within a few years of diagnosis.

Pemphigus vulgaris is also an autoimmune disease. In contrast to bullous pemphigoid, antidesmoglein antibodies are directed against the intercellular surfaces of epidermal keratinocytes (Bolognia 2008). Thus, cell-cell adhesion is disrupted, bullae break apart easily, and shallow erosions covered with crust are the usual clinical findings. Unlike bullous pemphigoid, pemphigus vulgaris is found in a younger population (patients usually in their thirties or forties). Lesions in pemphigus vulgaris usually start in the oral mucosa and then spread to the skin. Pemphigus vulgaris can involve the scalp, face, axilla, groin, trunk and points of pressure. These lesions are painful and less commonly itch. Nikolsky sign is also present, with easy skin removal by applying a slight shearing force on normal-appearing skin adjacent to the lesion.

Epidermolysis bullosa acquisita (EBA) is worth mentioning in the differential diagnosis of this patient because it shares some clinical and histological features of bullous pemphigoid. EBA is a chronic autoimmune disease characterized by severe subepidermal blistering, scars, and milia with a tendency to form in traumatized areas of the body. A specialized form of direct immunofluorescence on salt-split skin is required to differentiate between EBA and BP (Bolognia 2008).

Bullous scabies can mimic the histology and direct immunofluorescent findings of bullous pemphigoid and therefore must be included in the differential diagnosis (Shahab 2003). History and mineral oil mounted skin scrapings can inexpensively and rapidly make the appropriate diagnosis.

Based on the patient's medical history, clinical picture, and biopsy results, the diagnosis of bullous pemphigoid was made. Of note, direct immunofluorescent skin biopsies should be obtained from perilesional skin rather than intact blisters or erosions to have the best diagnostic sensitivity.

The patient was instructed to avoid sun exposure and keep the lesions dry and clean. Topical clobetasol cream and tetracycline 500 mg bid were prescribed with good results. If a flare occurs systemic immunosuppressives could be considered as a next step.

Key Points

- Bullous pemphigoid is an immunoblistering disease.
- Lesion distribution is often the inner thighs, flexor surfaces of the forearms, axillae, groin, lower legs and lower abdomen.

References

Abbas AK, Fausto N, Kumar V. Robbins and Cotran pathologic basis of disease. 7th ed. Philadelphia: The Curtis Center; 2005. p. 1260–2.

Bolognia J, Jorizzo JL, Rapini RP. Dermatology. St. Louis: Mosby/Elsevier; 2008.

Johnson RA, Suurmond D, Wolff K. Fitzpatrick's color atlas & synopsis of clinical dermatology. 5th ed. New York: McGraw-Hill; 2005. p. 100–8.

Shahab RK, Loo DS. Bullous Scabies. J Am Acad Dermatol. 2003 Aug; 49(2):346–350.

Chapter 2
67 Year Old with Multiple Nodules on the Thigh

A 67-year-old man presents with a 2–3-week history of an ulceration of the left ankle, accompanied by swelling of both legs. He also noted new painful lesions on his thigh and punched-out ulcers on the lower legs. A workup for deep vein thrombophlebitis was negative.

On examination, there were multiple red-to-violaceous deep dermal nodules on the right thigh. Both legs were edematous with scale and mild erythema.

Based on the case description and the photograph, what is your diagnosis?

1. Erythema nodosum
2. Superficial thrombophlebitis
3. Pyoderma gangrenosum
4. Polyarteritis nodosa

Diagnosis

Polyarteritis nodosa

R.A. Norman, J. Endo, *Clinical Cases in Geriatric Dermatology,* Clinical Cases in Dermatology, DOI 10.1007/978-1-4471-4135-8_2, © Springer-Verlag London 2013

Discussion

Polyarteritis is a multisystem vasculitis that can cause "punched out" skin ulceration, livedo reticularis, and inflammatory nodules on the thighs and elsewhere. The central nervous system, lungs, kidneys, gastrointestinal tract, and heart may be involved (Courtney et al., 2003; Cox et al., 2010; Goodless et al., 1990; Matteson 1999; Morgan et al., 2010). The patient was referred back to his internist for a workup for possible internal involvement and for systemic immunosuppressive therapy.

Diagnostic Pearls

Consider polyarteritis nodosa in a patient with new onset of painful nodules on the lower extremities associated with cutaneous ulcerations (Thomas et al., 1983).

Erythema nodosum produces multiple subcutaneous red tender nodules on the shins. However, it almost never causes leg ulcerations and does not have livedo.

Superficial thrombophlebitis can cause tender red nodules on the lower extremities but does not cause ulcers. Deep vein thrombophlebitis can lead to ulcerations but should not produce multiple nodules on the thighs.

Pyoderma gangrenosum can present with punched-out ulcers on the lower extremities and can begin with nodules. However, pyoderma gangrenosum rapidly ulcerates, often has significant periulcer erythema and undermining, is often associated with pathergy (pustule formation and skin breakdown with trivial skin trauma), lacks livedo changes, and heals with cribiform scarring.

Key Points

- Polyarteritis nodosa is a multisystem vasculitis that can cause "punched out" skin ulceration, livedo reticularis, and inflammatory nodules on the skin.

- Consider polyarteritis nodosa in a patient with new onset of painful nodules on the lower extremities associated with cutaneous ulcerations.

References

Courtney RH, Glenn GR. Polyarteritis nodosa and cutaneous polyarteritis nodosa. SKINmed: Dermatol Clini. 2003;2:277–86.

Cox N, Jorizzo JL, Bourke JF, Savage COS. Vasculitis, neutrophilic dermatoses and related disorders. In: Burns T, Breathnach S, Cox N, Griffiths C, editors. Rook's textbook of dermatology. 8th ed. Oxford, UK: Wiley-Blackwell; 2010.

Goodless DR, Dhawan SS, Alexis J, Wiszniak J. Cutaneous periarteritis nodosa. Int J Dermatol. 1990;29:611–5.

Matteson EL. A history of early investigation in polyarteritis nodosa. Arthritis Care Res. 1999;12:294–302.

Morgan AJ, Schwartz RA. Cutaneous polyarteritis nodosa: a comprehensive review. Int J Dermatol. 2010;49:750–6.

Thomas RM, Black MM. The wide clinical spectrum of polyarteritis nodosa with cutaneous involvement. Clin Exp Dermatol. 1983;8:47–59.

Chapter 3
Ulcer on the Hand of a 74 Year Old Woman

A 74 year old women presented with 4-month history of non-healing ulceration on the dorsal hand that had not responded to antibiotics (Fig. 3.1). Her past medical history includes rheumathoid arthritis.

Examination of the lesion revealed a solitary ulceration covered with dense eschar and perilesional erythema and an undermined border.

Based on the case description and the photograph, what is your diagnosis?

1. Squamous cell carcinoma
2. Rheumathoid vasculitis
3. Pyoderma gangrenosum (neutrophilic dermatosis of the dorsal hand)

Diagnosis

Pyoderma gangrenosum

R.A. Norman, J. Endo, *Clinical Cases in Geriatric Dermatology,* Clinical Cases in Dermatology, DOI 10.1007/978-1-4471-4135-8_3, © Springer-Verlag London 2013

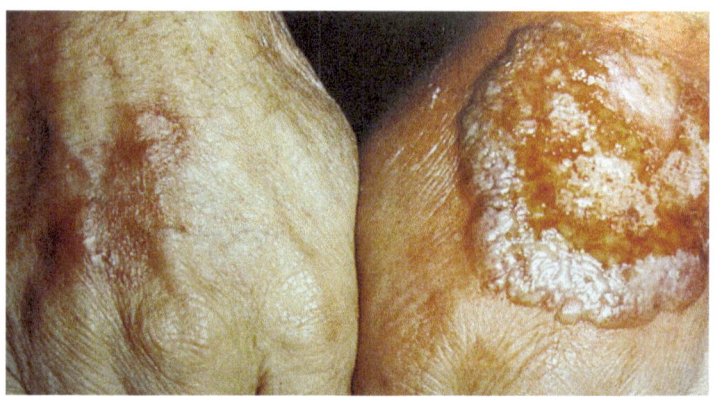

FIGURE 3.1   A 74 year old women with ulceration on the hands

Discussion

One should consider pyoderma gangrenosum in the differential of a patient who presents with a rapid skin ulcerations, undermined borders, and a history of autoimmune disorders including rheumatoid arthritis (Brooklyn et al., 2006; Conrad et al., 2005). Pyoderma granulosum is a diagnosis of exclusion, and biopsy is used to rule out other causes (Reichrath et al., 2005; Su et al., 2004; Su et al., 1986).

Squamous cell carcinoma rarely propagates this quickly. This tumor's borders are often raised and irregular.

Rheumathoid vasculitis can produce ulcerative lesions in patients suffering from rheumatoid arthritis, especially in those with high titers of rheumatoid factor. However, the ulcers produced in this condition lack undermined borders, cribiform scarring, and pathergy.

Key Points

- Pyoderma gangrenosum is an ulcerative process associated with other autoimmune diseases, such as rheumatoid arthritis and inflammatory bowel disease.
- Pyoderma gangrenosum is in the differential of a patient who presents with rapidly progressive skin ulcerations, undermined borders, and a history of autoimmune disorders.

References

Brooklyn T, Dunnill G, Probert C. Diagnosis and treatment of pyoderma gangrenosum. BMJ. 2006;333(7560):181–4.

Conrad C, Trüeb RM. Pyoderma gangrenosum. J Dtsch Dermatol Ges. 2005;3:334–42.

Reichrath J, Bens G, Bonowitz A, Tilgen W. Treatment recommendations for pyoderma gangrenosum: an evidence-based review of the literature based on more than 350 patients. J Am Acad Dermatol. 2005;53(2):273–83.

Su WPD, Davis MDP, Weenig RH, Powell FC, Perry HO. Pyoderma gangrenosum: clinicopathologic correlation and proposed diagnostic criteria. Int J Dermatol. 2004;43:790–800.

Su WPD, Sctiroeter AL, Perry HO, Powell FC. Histopathologic and immunopathologic study of pyoderma gangrenosum. J Cutan Pathol. 1986;13:323–30.

Chapter 4
Elderly Man with Rash on Chest and Back

A 64-year-old male with a rash on his back. His medical history was notable for a previous diagnosis of "lupus" a decade ago. He denied taking any medications. Physical exam revealed a well-developed, well-nourished, male without malar rash who had several scaly, annular plaques on his chest and back (Fig. 4.1).

Based on the case description and the photograph, what is your diagnosis?

1. Nummular eczema
2. Subacute cutaneous lupus erythematosus
3. Psoriasis
4. Sarcoidosis
5. Granuloma annulare

Diagnosis

Subacute cutaneous lupus erythematosus

R.A. Norman, J. Endo, *Clinical Cases in Geriatric Dermatology,* Clinical Cases in Dermatology, DOI 10.1007/978-1-4471-4135-8_4, © Springer-Verlag London 2013

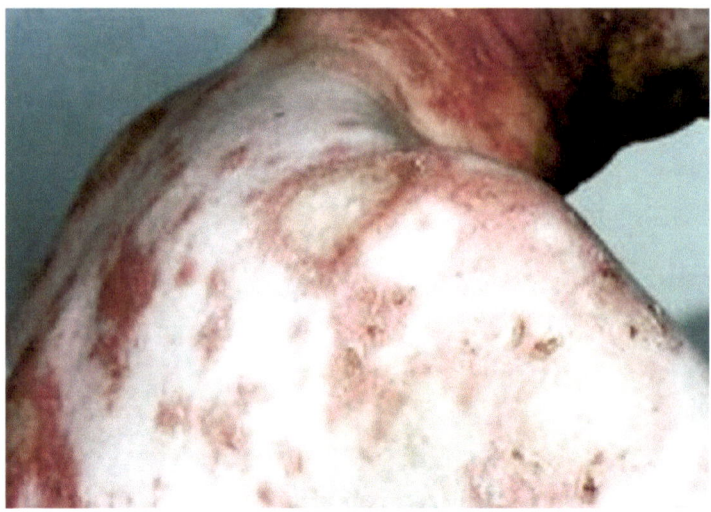

FIGURE 4.1   A 64-year-old male presented with several annular, scaly plaques on his chest and back

Discussion

Skin biopsy showed hyperkeratosis, atrophy, focal liquefaction of the epidermis and perivascular and perifollicular infiltration of lymphocytes and histiocytes. Alcian blue stain revealed copious mucin in the dermis. Lupus serologies, renal function, complete blood counts, and urinalysis were all normal.

If cutaneous lupus is suspected, a drug-induced lupus should first be excluded. Up to one-third of cases of SCLE are drug-induced and potentially reversible by medication cessation (Grönhagen 2012). An exhaustive list of causative drugs have been published (Lowe 2011). Next, systemic involvement (systemic lupus erythematosus) should be excluded. Several caveats should be noted with systemic lupus evaluation. Firstly, antinuclear antibodies (ANA) are sensitive for lupus but are not specific. That is, other autoimmune conditions or even advanced age can lead to false positive results (Bolognia 2008). Secondly, some patients with SCLE will progress to develop systemic disease, perhaps at least 10%. However, the reported figures are highly variable among studies (Bolognia 2008, Grönhagen 2011).

In the absence of systemic involvement or medication-induced etiology, SCLE is often managed with topical steroids and antimalarials. Patients must meticuously avoid the sun or use broad-spectrum sunblock. In refractory cases, other systemic immunosuppressives can be considered (Bolognia 2008).

Key Points

- Subacute cutaneous lupus erythematosus (SCLE) presents as photosensitive, non-scarring, scaly violaceous plaques.
- SCLE may be drug-induced, and thorough review of medications to search for culprits must be performed.
- A subset of SCLE patients can develop systemic lupus erythematosus (SLE). Thus, appropriate laboratory monitoring is important.

References

Rahman A, Isenberg DA. Review article: systemic lupus erythematosus. N Engl J Med. 2008;358(9):929–39.

Bolognia J, Jorizzo JL, Rapini RP. Dermatology. St. Louis: Mosby/Elsevier; 2008.

Goodfield MJD, Jones SK, Veale DJ. The 'connective tissue diseases'. In: Burns T, Breathnach S, Cox N, Griffiths C, editors. Rook's textbook of dermatology. 8th ed. Oxford: Wiley-Blackwell; 2010.

Grönhagen CM, Fored CM, Granath F, Nyberg F. Cutaneous lupus erythematosus and the association with systemic lupus erythematosus: a population-based cohort of 1088 patients in Sweden. Br J Dermatol. 2011;164(6):1335–41.

Grönhagen CM, Fored CM, Linder M, Granath F, Nyberg F. HYPERLINK "/pubmed/22458771" Subacute cutaneous lupus erythematosus and its association with drugs: a population-based matched case–control study of 234 patients in Sweden. Br J Dermatol. 2012;167(2):296–305.

James W, Berger T, Elston D. Andrews' diseases of the skin: clinical dermatology. 10th ed. Philadelphia: Saunders; 2005.

Lowe G, Henderson CL, Grau RH, Hansen CB, Sontheimer RD. A systematic review of drug-induced subacute cutaneous lupus erythematosus. Br J Dermatol. 2011; 164(3): 465–472.

Weinstein C, Miller MH, Axtens R, Littlejohn GO, Dorevitch AP, Buchanan R. Lupus and non-lupus cutaneous manifestations in systemic lupus erythematosus. Aust N Z J Med. 1987;17:501–6.

Part II
Infestations

Chapter 5
78 Year Old Man with Severe Pruritus

During a nursing home visit, a 78 year old man reported severe itching, worse at night.

Examination showed excoriated nodules on the penis, scrotum, axillae, waist, buttocks, and chest (Fig. 5.1).

Based on the case description and the photograph, what is your diagnosis?

1. Dermatitis herpetiformis
2. Scabies
3. Prurigo nodularis
4. Papular urticaria

Diagnosis

Scabies

Discussion

Scabies is a pruritic and contagious infestation of the skin caused by the *Sarcoptes scabiei* mite (Hicks et al. 2009; Makigami et al. 2011).

R.A. Norman, J. Endo, *Clinical Cases in Geriatric Dermatology*, Clinical Cases in Dermatology, DOI 10.1007/978-1-4471-4135-8_5, © Springer-Verlag London 2013

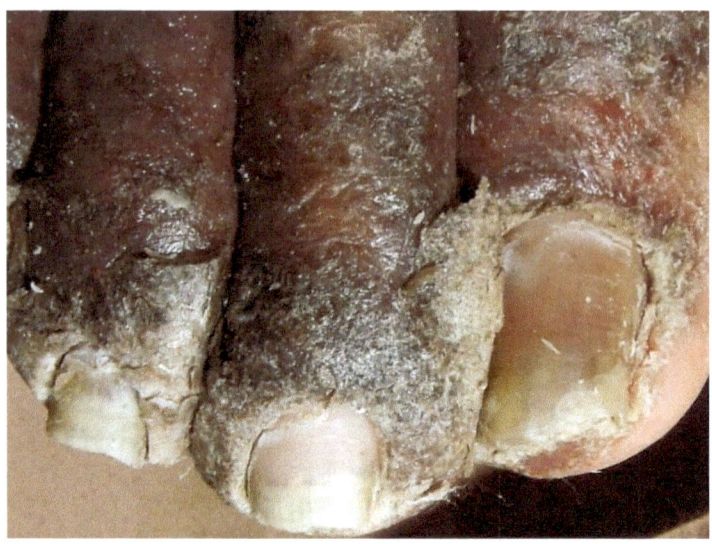

Figure 5.1 Excoriated nodules

The institutional risk factors for scabies among nursing homes include institution (over 30 years old), size greater than 120 beds, and resident population to health care workers exceeding 10:1 (Chosidow 2000).

The classic clinical exam finding are linear or serpiginous burrows or scattered papules. Affected areas often include the interdigital web spaces, wrists, axillae, genitals, and breasts. In immunocompromised patients, crusted (formerly termed "Norwegian") scabies presents as lichenified, generalized eczematous plaques.

Diagnosis of scabies is rapidly confirmed by collecting skin scrapings from multiple affected sites and mounting on mineral oil glass slide. The mites are not always present, so the clinician must be able to also identify the feces (scybala) or eggs of the mite (Bolognia 2008).

Treatment should be recommended for not only the individual patient, but also for any co-inhabitants due to the contagious nature of scabies. Linens and clothing should be treated with a machine dryer on a high-heat setting, otherwise placed in a sealed bag for at least 3 days. Living quarters must be decontaminated.

The first-line therapy is typically topical 5% permethrin cream applied from the neck down once, left on overnight, then repeated 1 week later to ensure eradication of mites that might be in different stages of its life cycle. All lesions should be healed within 4 weeks after the treatment, though the patient should be counseled pruritus can last for several weeks even after successful treatment. Nonetheless, re-infestations can occur.

Oral ivermectin (150–200 ug/kg) is an alternative treatment. One comparative study found that two doses of ivermectin was better than a single permethrin application. One potential advantage of ivermectin over permethrin, particularly in the institutional setting, is the labor and time cost-savings of oral medication over topical applications. In community-dwelling patients with cognitive or mobility difficulties, oral application might also be a reasonable alternative (Sharma et al. 2011; Strong et al. 2011).

Two major complications of scabetic infestation are worth noting. The severe pruritus associated with scabies can be treated with either topical or oral glucocortiocsteroids; or low doses of oral antihistamines. It is also important to identify and treat secondary impetiginization of gram positive organisms with either topical mupirocin or oral anti-infectives.

Key Points

- Scabies is a contagious infestation caused by the Sarcoptes scabiei mite that can present with burrows, papules, or generalized eczematous crusting.
- Treatment involves decontamination of linens, clothing, and living quarters as well as medical therapy of the patient and all co-inhabitants.
- Nursing homes, especially older or high-volume institutions, can be at particularly high risk for epidemics.

References

Bolognia J, Jorizzo JL, Rapini RP. Dermatology. St. Louis: Mosby/ Elsevier; 2008.

Chosidow O, Scabies and pediculosis. Lancet 2000;355(9206): 819–26.

Hicks MI, Elston DM. Scabies. Dermatol Ther. 2009;22:279–92.

Makigami K, Ohtaki N, Ishii N, Tamashiro T, Yoshida S, Yasumura S. Risk factors for recurrence of scabies: a retrospective study of scabies patients in a long-term care hospital. J Dermatol. 2011;38(9):874–9.

Sharma R, Singal A. Topical permethrin and oral ivermectin in the management of scabies: a prospective, randomized, double blind, controlled study. Indian J Dermatol Venereol Leprol. 2011;77(5):581–6.

Strong M, Johnstone P. Cochrane review: interventions for treating scabies. Evidence-Based Child Health: Cochrane Rev J. 2011;6: 1790–862.

Chapter 6
A 62 Year Old with Painful Blisters on the Face

A 62 year old man reported with a 2-day history of facial itching and burning. Exam showed grouped vesicles on an erythematous base, confined to a distinct dermatome and not crossing the midline (Figs. 6.1, 6.2, and 6.3).

Based on the case description and the photograph, what is your diagnosis?

1. Herpes simplex
2. Herpes zoster
3. Cellulitis
4. Contact dermatitis

Diagnosis

Herpes zoster

Discussion

Herpes zoster also known as shingles, is caused by re-activation of the varicella zoster virus within a previously infected dorsal root ganglion. It generally afflicts older adults or immuno-compromised individuals immunocompromised adult. The

R.A. Norman, J. Endo, *Clinical Cases in Geriatric Dermatology*, Clinical Cases in Dermatology,
DOI 10.1007/978-1-4471-4135-8_6,
© Springer-Verlag London 2013

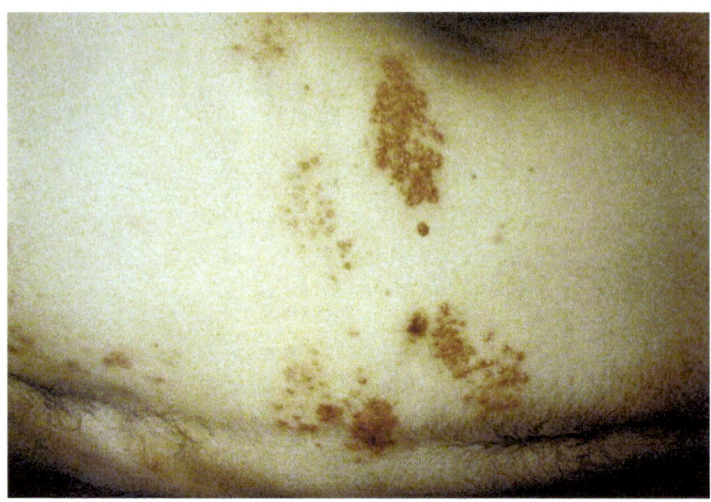

FIGURE 6.1 A 62 year old man with itching and burning on face

practitioner should be suspicious of an underlying lymphoma, leukemia, or Acquired Immunodeficiency Syndrome (AIDS).

The onset of cutaneous herpes zoster is usually preceded by a 1–3 day prodrome of pain or paresthesias in the affected dermatome. In some cases of thoracic involvement, the pain of zoster can mimic cardiac angina. Subsequently, erythematous papules, pustules and vesicles (sometimes hemorrhagic or crusted) in the same distribution appear.

Herpes zoster sometimes presents in multiple contiguous or noncontiguous dermatomes (zoster multiplex). There may be small islands of lesions at a distant location. Disseminated zoster rarely occurs.

The most common complication is postherpetic neuralgia, which is defined as chronic pain or neuropathic symptoms that persist after resolution of the rash. Risk factors include older age, severity of acute and prodromal pain. Other postherpetic

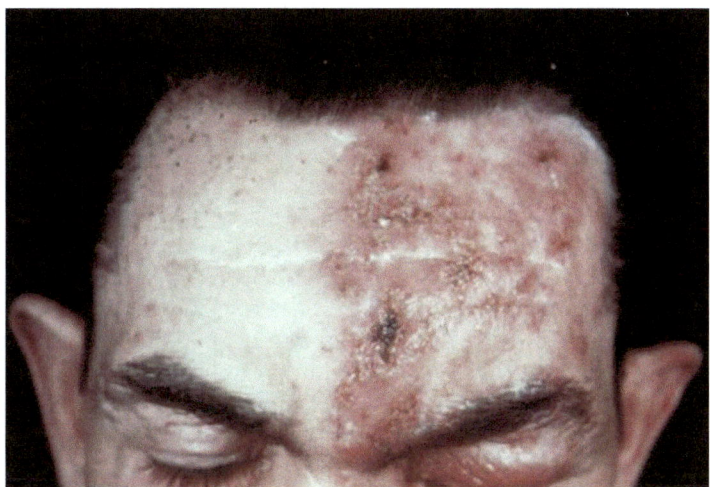

FIGURE 6.2 A 62 year old man with itching and burning on face

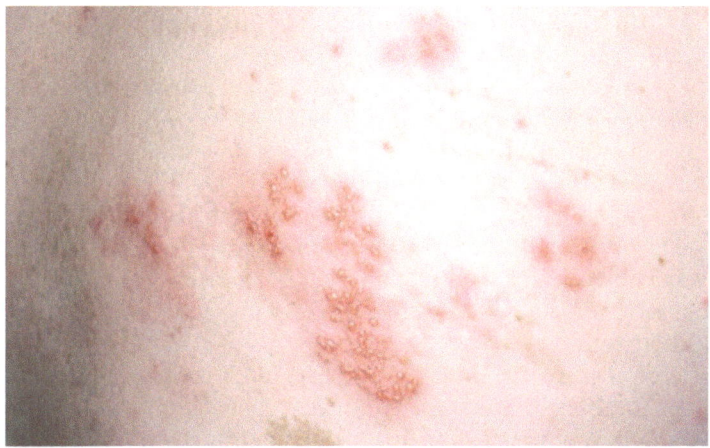

FIGURE 6.3 Grouped vesicles on an erythematous base, confined to a distinct dermatome and not crossing the midline

peripheral motor neuropathies include peripheral motor neuropathies, neurogenic bladder, and diaphragmatic paralysis. They are usually transient (Assefzadah 2010). Another dreaded complication is herpes zoster ophthalmicus. This occurs in 10–25 % of zoster cases and can cause blindness.

Immunocompromised Patient Considerations

There is an increased incidence of herpes zoster in immunocompromised persons, such as cancer patients, transplant recipients, and those taking immunosuppressants. Episodes of herpes zoster tend to be more extensive and longer lasting in these populations. Furthermore, the clinical presentation can be atypical, with disseminated or generalized herpes zoster, multiple recurrences, systemic infection with visceral dissemination, and CNS involvement have been reported (Madkan et al. 2008; Tyring 2007).

Diagnosis, Prevention & Management

The quickest and least expensive diagnostic test is the Tzanck smear. Direct fluorescent antigen (DFA), viral culture, or polymerase chain reaction (PCR) can be useful.

The Centers for Disease Control (CDC) recommends a live attenuated zoster vaccine for patients aged 50 and older (Harpaz et al. 2008). Notable contraindications for the vaccine include the actively immunocompromised, allergy to gelatin or neomycin, and those with active tuberculosis infection.

Oral acyclovir should be administered within the first 72 h of acute zoster symptom onset (Dworkin et al. 2007). Postherpetic neuralgia can be challenging to manage (Bowsher 1997; Decroix et al. 2000). Options are numerous and can include non-steroidal anti-inflammatory drugs, opioids or tricyclic antidepressants (Plaghki et al. 2004).

Key Points

- Herpes zoster is caused by reactivation of the varicella zoster virus within dorsal root ganglia.
- The clinical presentation can vary, particularly in immuno-compromised populations.
- Vaccination to prevent zoster and its dreaded complications (especially postherpetic neuralgia) are recommended for adults aged 50 years and older.

References

Assefzadeh M, Ghasemi R, Naimian SH, Shahali H, Sajadi E. A 72 year-old diabetic woman with herpes zoster paresis: a case report. Iranian Journal of Clinical Infectious Diseases 2010;5(4): 239–241.

Bowsher D. The effects of pre-emptive treatment of postherpetic neuralgia with amitriptyline: a randomized, double-blind, placebo-controlled trial. J Pain Symptom Manage. 1997;13(6):327–31.

Decroix J, Paetsch H, Gonzalez R, et al. Factors influencing pain outcome in herpes zoster: an observational study with valaciclovir. Valaciclovir International Zoster Assessment Group (VIZA). J Eur Acad Dermatol Venereol. 2000;14(1):23–33.

Dworkin RH, Johnson RW, Breuer J, et al. Recommendations for the management of herpes zoster. Clin Infect Dis. 2007;44 Suppl 1:51–526.

Harpaz R, Ortega-Sanchez R, Seward JF, Advisory Committee on Immunization Practices (ACIP) Centers for Disease Control and Prevention (CDC). Prevention of herpes zoster: recommendations of the Advisory Committee on Immunization Practices (ACIP). MMWR Recomm Rep. 2008;57(RR-S):1–30. quiz CE2-4.

Madkan V, Sea K, Brantley J, et al. Human herpesviruses. In: Bolognia J, Iorizao J, Rapini RP, editors. Dermatology. 2nd ed. St. Louis, MO: Mosby; 2008. p. 1204–8.

Plaghki L, Adriaensen H, Morlion B, et al. Systematic overview of the pharmacological management of postherpetic neuralgia. An evaluation of the clinical value of critically selected drug treatments based on efficacy and safety outcomes from randomized controlled studies. Dermatology. 2004;208(3):206–16.

Tyring SK. Management of herpes zoster and postherpetic neuralgia. J Am Acad Dermatol. 2007;S7(6 Suppl):S136–42.

Chapter 7
70-Year Old Man with Oval Macules

A 70 year old man presented to our office with itchy discoloration on his neck and upper trunk that was worse in the summer. He had reddish-brown reticulated macules coaslesced into larger patches with minimal scaling (Figs. 7.1 and 7.2).

Based on the case description and the photographs, what is your diagnosis?

1. Tinea corporis
2. Psoriasis
3. Vitiligo
4. Small plaque parapsoriasis
5. Tinea versicolor

Diagnosis

Tinea versicolor

R.A. Norman, J. Endo, *Clinical Cases in Geriatric Dermatology,* Clinical Cases in Dermatology, DOI 10.1007/978-1-4471-4135-8_7, © Springer-Verlag London 2013

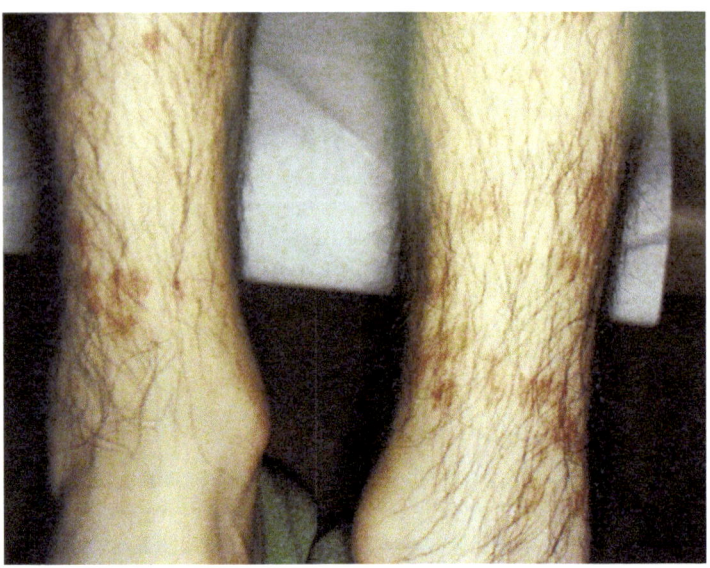

FIGURE 7.1 A plethora of reddish-brown round macules that were minimally scaly

Discussion

Tinea versicolor is a superficial fungal infection that is caused by the organism *Malassezia furfur. M. furfur* is a normal resident of human flora; however, under certain conditions, such as heat and humidity, it can become pathological (Hay et al. 2008; Rapini et al. 2007; Reiss et al. 2011). The name of the condition describes the fact that the lesions can vary in color, from white (hypopigmentation) to reddish-brown. The most common location is the neck and upper trunk. Diagnosis is confirmed with potassium hydroxide (KOH) skin scraping, which demonstrates the dimorphic "spaghetti and meatballs" yeast.

The patient was treated with ketoconazole 400 mg, given in two doses over 1 week. The eruption resolved completely. One therapeutic pearl is to have the patient break out into a sweat shortly after taking ketoconazole, which increases skin

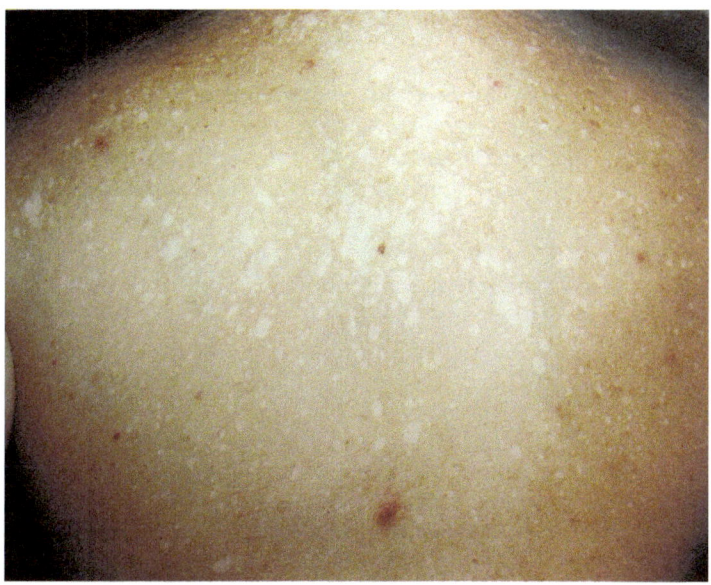

FIGURE 7.2 A plethora of white and tan round macules that were minimally scaly

bioavailability of the medication (Zaias 1989). Patients should be counseled that the discoloration can take months to resolve even after successful treatment.

Tinea corporis is caused by dermatophytes and typically are red scaly plaques on the trunk and neck. Unlike tinea versicolor, tinea corporis is often annular and not polycyclic. The typical KOH preparation shows long, branching hyphae with septae.

Psoriasis usually causes scaly red papules and plaques that are often discrete and favors flexor surfaces of extremities, buttocks, and the umbilicus. It produces extremely thick scaling lesions that are often red in color, not brown.

Vitiligo often affects the orifices of the body, bony prominences, hands, feet, and genitals. It is characterized by complete depigmentation under Wood's lamp and does not have scale.

Small plaque parapsoriasis most often presents as scaly patches that do not coalesce to the same extent as tinea versicolor.

Key Points

- Tinea versicolor is a superficial fungal infection that is caused by the organism Malassezia furfur.
- Diagnosis is confirmed with potassium hydroxide skin scraping, which demonstrates the dimorphic "spaghetti and meatballs".
- Discoloration can take many months to fade well after successful treatment completion.

References

Hay RJ, Moore MK. Mycology. In: Burns T, Breathnach S, Cox N, Griffiths C, editors. Rook's textbook of dermatology. 7th ed. Malden: Blackwell Publishing, Inc.; 2008.

Rapini Ronald P, Bolognia Jean L, Jorizzo Joseph L. Dermatology: 2-Volume Set. St. Louis: Mosby; 2007. Chapter 76.

Reiss E, Shadomy HJ, Lyon GM. Dermatomycoses, in fundamental medical mycology. Hoboken: Wiley; 2011.

Zaias N. Pityriasis versicolor with ketoconazole. J Am Acad Dermatol. 1989;20(4):703.

Chapter 8
68 Year Old with Anogenital Lesions

A 68 year old with a 15-year history of human immuno-deficiency virus (HIV) stated he had not been compliant with his HIV medications over the last year and developed cauliflower-like vegetative red-brown papules on his genitals and gluteal cleft (Figs. 8.1 and 8.2).

Based on the case description and the photograph, what is your diagnosis?

1. Condylomata lata of secondary syphilis
2. Condyloma accuminata
3. Bowen's disease
4. Lichen planus

Diagnosis

Condyloma accuminata

Discussion

Warts (verrucae) can be spread by scratching or other trauma. Several variants exist:

R.A. Norman, J. Endo, *Clinical Cases in Geriatric Dermatology,* Clinical Cases in Dermatology, DOI 10.1007/978-1-4471-4135-8_8, © Springer-Verlag London 2013

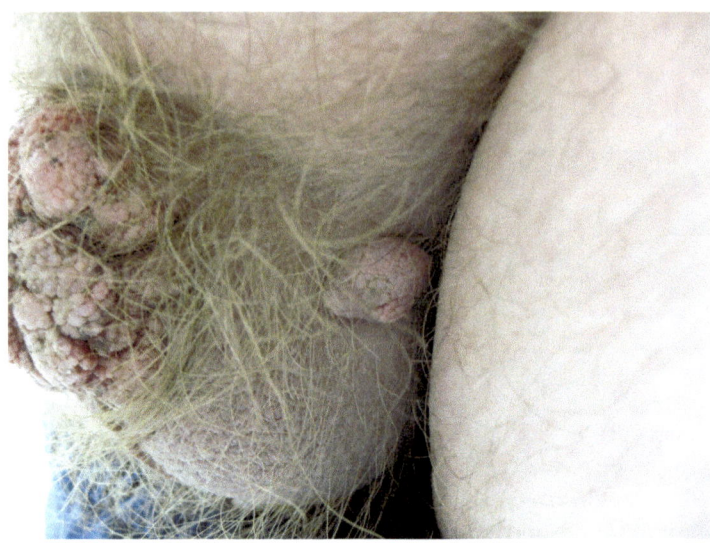

FIGURE 8.1 68 year old with a 15-year history of HIV stated he had not been compliant with his HIV medications over the last year and had developed cauliflower-like vegetative red-brown papules on his genitals and gluteal cleft

1. Flat warts: flat-topped, small, flesh-colored papules on the face, dorsal hands, and legs
2. Filiform (filamentous) warts: pedunculated lesions often on the neck, lip, eyelid
3. Papular, exophytic, "common" warts: large, verrucous plaques on the fingers, hands
4. Mosaic endophytic warts: plantar warts.

No uniformly successful preventive or treatment measures exist. The following may be tried (Fox et al. 2005):

1. Surgery-paring, extraction. The patient should be cautioned regarding possible scarring, recurrence, and discomfort.
2. Topical keratolytics- salicylic acid.
3. Vesicants-cantharidin (Cantharone) is highly caustic and difficult to obtain in the United States.

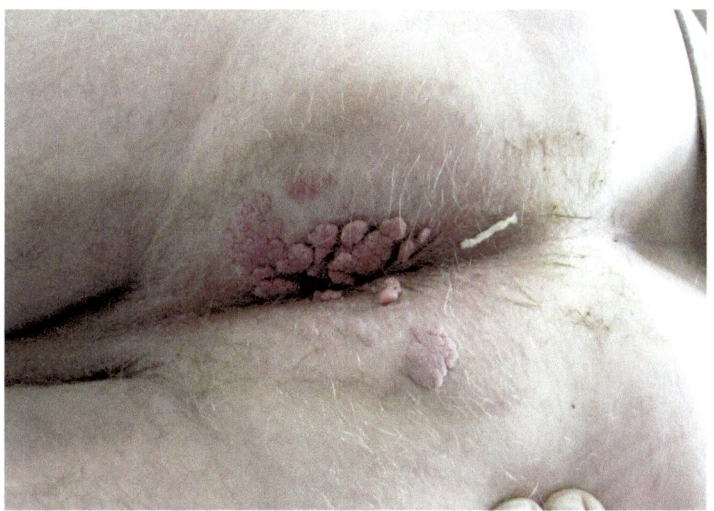

FIGURE 8.2 Cauliflower-like vegetative red-brown papules on his genitals and gluteal cleft

4. Colposcopy followed by laser eradication of genital warts can be considered.
5. Liquid nitrogen cryotherapy is simple and effective. But it is also painful and can produce a ring of warts around the treatment site.
6. Interferon or bleomycin can be effective, but are also expensive, inconsistent in curing verruca, and have significant side effects (Reichman et al. 1988).
7. Topical immunomodulation: imiqumod.
8. Sinecatechins (marketed as Veregen and Polyphenon E) are extracted from green tea and other components. It might cause less irritation than other treatments (Meltzer et al. 2009).

Warts are caused by human papilloma virus (HPV) infection. Some HPV types cause cervical dysplasia and cancer in women and bowenoid papulosis and squamous cell cancer of the penis in men. Many warts resolve spontaneously, but some are stubbornly recurrent. On occasion, biopsy can be considered to rule out verrucous squamous cell carcinoma, particularly in immunosuppressed patients.

Gardasil (Merck & Co.) is a vaccine that protects against human papillomavirus types 16, 18, 6, and 11. Types 6 and 11 cause genital warts, while 16 and 18 cause cervical cancer. The vaccine is preventive, not therapeutic. The vaccine is approved for use by young women and men.

Differentials condylomata lata of secondary syphilis are broader (lata) and less pointed (acuminata).

Bowen's disease is squamous cell carcinoma in situ and is not generally this large, elevated, and verrucous. Often it appears as an inflamed patch or thin plaque. Larger lesions can reach several centimeters in diameter.

Lichen planus is a pruritic, papular eruption characterized by its violaceous color, polygonal shape, and lacy white appearance (Wickham's striae). Lichen planus is often also found on the wrists and sometimes genitalia or oral mucosa.

Key Points

- Condyloma accuminata is caused by human papilloma virus (HPV) infection.
- Certain types of HPV are considered "high risk" for evolving into dysplasia or squamous cell carcinoma.
- Condyloma accuminata is a common manifestation in HIV, often occurring in unusual locations.

References

Fox PA, Tung MY. Human papillomavirus: burden of illness and treatment cost considerations. Am J Clin Dermatol. 2005;6(6):365–81.

Meltzer SM, Monk BJ, Tewari KS. Green tea catechins for treatment of external genital warts. Am J Obstet Gynecol. 2009;200(3):233.

Reichman RC, Oakes O, Bonnez W, et al. Treatment of condyloma acuminatum with-three different interferons administered intralesionally. A double-blind, placebo-controlled trial. Ann Intern Med. 1988;108:675–9.

Chapter 9
72 Year Old Male with Diffuse Rash

A 72 year old male seen in the nursing home presented with an eruption of bright, 'beefy' red erythema involving his back, buttocks and legs (Fig. 9.1). The rash was surrounded by satellite pustules and papules located at the periphery. Some areas were eroded, raw, and oozing. The patient had a history of diabetes, and a 15-year history of steroid use for chronic obstructive pulmonary disease (COPD).

Based on the case description and the photograph, what is your diagnosis?

1. Eczema
2. Cellulitis
3. Tinea corporis
4. Candidiasis
5. Psoriasis

Diagnosis

Candidiasis

R.A. Norman, J. Endo, *Clinical Cases in Geriatric Dermatology,* Clinical Cases in Dermatology, DOI 10.1007/978-1-4471-4135-8_9, © Springer-Verlag London 2013

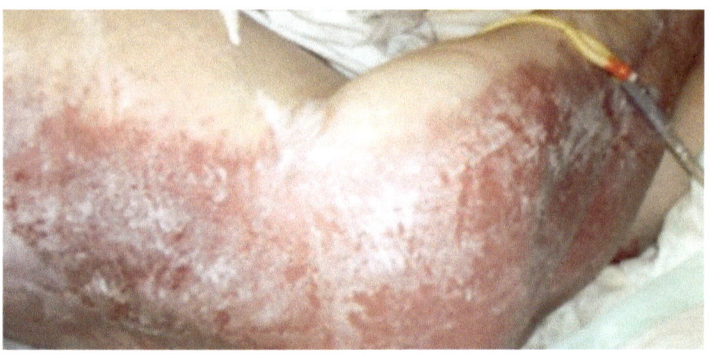

FIGURE 9.1 A 72 year old male presented with an eruption of bright, 'beefy' red erythema involving his back, buttocks and legs

Discussion

Fungal infections are commonly seen in the older population. There are three groups main organisms that cause cutaneous fungal infections: dermatophytes (noninvasive and only grow on superficial layers of skin), yeasts (e.g., candida), and non-dermatophyte molds (Elewski et al. 1989; James et al. 2006). Of note, dermatophytes do not grow on routine fungal culture media and require special temperature and medium. Potassium hydroxide (KOH) examination should be considered on scaling eruptions to look for dermatophytosis.

Candidiasis is an infection caused by yeast, often of the species *Candida albicans*. Infection may occur on this skin, in mucous membranes, or the nails. Candidiasis of the oral cavity is called *thrush*. Infection at the base of the nails is called *paronychia*.

Candida albicans is normal flora on human skin. Breaks in the skin allow penetration of the yeast into the skin and infection occurs, particularly if the patient has predisposing conditions: diabetes mellitus, obesity, heat, chronic debilitation, altered immune status (AIDS), chronic antibiotic use, or long-term systemic steroid therapy (Pappas 1998).

The form most commonly seen in the older population is *intertriginous candidiasis,* which affects moist body fold, including the inguinal, inframammary, infraabdominal, and axillary folds. The infection caused by the yeast ranges from superficial lesions to disseminated infections. Widespread, or disseminated, infection is more commonly seen in immunocompromised individuals.

The patient may complain of pruritus and a burning sensation on the skin where the *Candidiasis* infection is present. The eruption often presents as bright, 'beefy' red erythema and is often surrounded by pustules and papules. Remnants of pustules may appear as macules with a scaly border.

Treatment

Topical treatments with nystatin, econazole, or imidaole are is often used when small areas are affected. Some over-the-counter products (e.g., clotrimazole, naftifine, terbinafine) are commonly stocked in skilled nursing facilities and often work well to clear the infection. Systemic therapy with oral or intravenous medications may be used for widespread infections (Lesher et al. 1987). These medications may affect prothrombin time (PT) levels in patients taking warfarin (Coumadin). Additional testing of this lab value may be ordered by the practitioner.

Differentials

Irritation or erythema under the breasts or the axilla does not always indicate a yeast infection. Sometimes skin breakdown from moisture and mechanical shearing in the absence of infection may cause *irritant intertrigo.* This does not require treatment with antifungal medications, but is best treated by keeping the area clean and dry and generous application of barrier creams (e.g., zinc oxide, petrolatum).

Differentials: Psoriasis can cause discrete scaly red papules and plaques. The scale is typically much thicker and satellite pustules or papules are absent.

Tinea corporis causes scaly red plaques that can occur on the trunk and neck. However, the lesions are often annular, rather than being the confluence of many small scaly macules.

Cellulitis is commonly caused by gram positive bacteria and typically presents with poorly demarcated erythema, swelling, pain, and warmth of the skin. Regional lymph nodes may also be enlarged and tender.

Eczema is typically accompanied by erythema, skin edema, crusting of the skin, and blisters that often show signs of cracking and ooze fluid.

Key Points

- Commonly caused by moisture, especially in the intertrigionous areas
- May be widespread, especially in immunocompromised persons
- Not all redness seen in intertriginous areas is Candidiasis. It may be caused by irritation (irritant intertrigo).

References

Elewski BE, Hazen PG. The superficial mycoses and the dermatophytes. J Am Acad Dermatol. 1989;21:655.

James WD, Berger TG et al. Andrews' diseases of the skin: clinical dermatology. Philadelphia: Saunders Elsevier; 2006.

Lesher J, Smith Jr JG. Antifungal agents in dermatology. J Am Acad Dermatol. 1987;17:383–94.

Pappas AA, Ray TL: Cutaneous and disseminated skin manifestations of candidiasis. In: Elewski BE, ed. Cutaneous Fungal Infections, 2nd edn. Massachusetts: Blackwell Science; 1998:91–117.

Part III
Premalignant Lesions and Neoplasms

Chapter 10
Growing Lesion on the Scalp

An 85 year-old African-American female patient presented to the office asking for evaluation of a skin lesion on her scalp (Fig. 10.1). It began as a small red lump about a year and a half ago experiencing a fall. Since then, it has been growing steadily to 10 cm in diameter. The patient denied prior treatment for the lesion. She was not taking medications and her past medical history was unremarkable.

Based on the case description and the photograph, what is your diagnosis?

1. Pyogenic granuloma
2. Angiosarcoma
3. Malignant melanoma
4. Fibrosarcoma

Diagnosis

Angiosarcoma

R.A. Norman, J. Endo, *Clinical Cases in Geriatric Dermatology,* Clinical Cases in Dermatology, DOI 10.1007/978-1-4471-4135-8_10, © Springer-Verlag London 2013

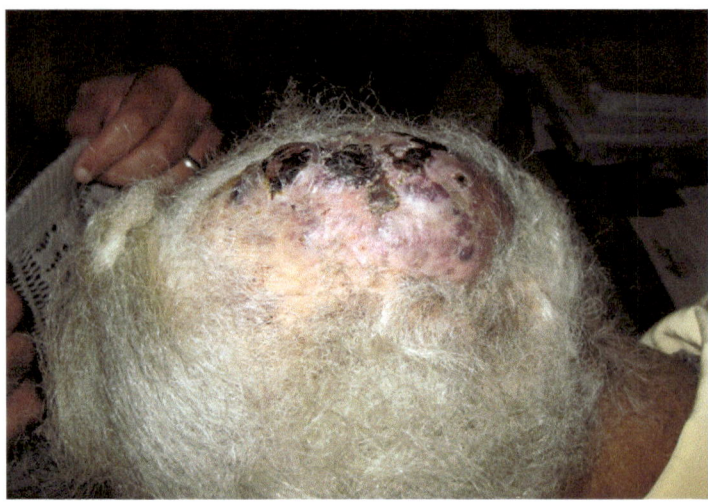

FIGURE 10.1 An 85 year-old African-American female patient presented for evaluation of a lesion on her scalp

Discussion

Angiosarcomas are classified as aggressive, vascular, soft tissue tumors that most often arise on the scalp and neck (Fakih et al. 2001). The two major forms of angiosarcomas are lymphedema-related (Stewart-Treves) vs non-lymphedema-related (Pawlik et al. 2003). There is a reddish-blue discoloration, and nodules and plaques may also be present. Sometimes the tumors can ulcerate, causing extensive bleeding due to its high vascularity. Although our patient presented with a single lesion, 50 % of patients have multiple lesions surgical. These tumors can metastasize – most often to the lung, regional lymph nodes, liver, and other areas of the skin. Angiosarcomas can recur in as many as 50% of cases.

Surgical resection is first-line treatment, especially with low-grade tumors (Lydiatt et al. 1994). No treatment has been consistently successful with high grade angiosarcomas. Due its ability to spread extensively through the scalp, achieving clear margins is often difficult. Postoperative radiation therapy, coupled with doxorubicin, may lead to better survival rates, especially when used in conjunction with surgery.

The most important prognostic factor, seems to be size of the tumor at initial diagnosis. Patients with tumor size less than 5 cm had better overall survival rates perhaps as high as 43 % (Holden et al. 1987).

Pyogenic granuloma appear as firm nodules and are usually red in color. They are dome shaped, may be sessile or pedunculated, and often have a collarette.

Malignant melanoma is a cancerous growth of melanocytes (pigment cells) that is diagnosed by biopsy.

Fibrosarcomas are large tumors that can penetrate to fascia.

Key Points

- Angiosarcomas are aggressive vascular soft tissue tumors that most often arise on the scalp and neck.
- Surgical excision is the treatment of choice, although recurrences are extremely high.

References

Fakih MG, Defrances MC, Paul Ohori N, Ramanathan RK. Unusual tumors involving the head and neck region – angiosarcoma of the scalp. J Clin Oncol. 2001;19(2):4173–4.

Holden CA, Spittle MF, Jones EW. Angiosarcoma of the face and scalp, prognosis and treatment. Cancer. 1987;59(5):1046–57.

Lydiatt WM, Shaha AR, Shah JP. Angiosarcoma of the head and neck. Am J Surg. 1994;168(5):451–4.

Pawlik TM, Paulino AF, Mcginn CJ, Baker LH, Cohen DS, Morris JS, Rees R, Sondak VK. Cutaneous angiosarcoma of the scalp. Cancer. 2003;98:1716–26.

Chapter 11
Questionable "Rash" on Right Leg

This is the case of a 74 year old man who had initially came in for a consult for what he described as a 3-week "rash" on his right leg (Fig. 11.1). At the time, the patient was experiencing dryness, irritation, itching, and redness on the affected area. He expressed symptoms of fatigue and low energy, but noted no decrease in appetite. Exam revealed masses that were firm to palpation. He denied trauma to the area. He was not on any medications.

Based on the case description and the photograph, what is your diagnosis?

1. Hodgkin disease
2. Cutaneous B-cell lymphoma
3. Anaplastic large cell lymphoma
4. Cutaneous manifestation of metastatic carcinoma

Diagnosis

Anaplastic large cell lymphoma (Stage IIE)

R.A. Norman, J. Endo, *Clinical Cases in Geriatric Dermatology,* Clinical Cases in Dermatology, DOI 10.1007/978-1-4471-4135-8_11, © Springer-Verlag London 2013

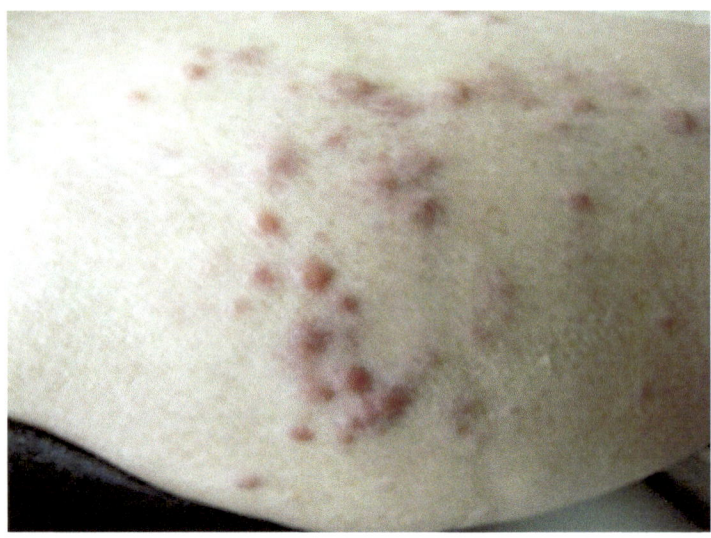

Figure 11.1 A 74 year old man presented with what he described as a 3-week "rash" on his right leg

Discussion

Anaplastic large cell lymphoma is a rare and highly aggressive form of non-Hodgkin lymphoma (NHL). The lymphoma is typically composed of T-lymphocytes and often presents at later stages with systemic symptoms such as early satiety, fatigue, or night sweats. The cause of anaplastic large cell lymphoma is unclear (Stein et al. 2000; Swerdlow et al. 2008).

In this case study, Stage II designates that the affected groups of lymph nodes are confined to only one side of the diaphragm. The letter "E" further classifies the lymphoma as extranodal, since it presented only on the skin.

Typically, patients suffering from anaplastic large cell lymphoma first notice a painless area of inflammation located in the neck, armpit or groin. The lymphoma can affect other organs such as the skin, lungs, liver, and bone marrow. Multiple groups of nodes are typically involved.

A diagnosis is made by performing a biopsy on an enlarged lymph node. If the patient displays a primary cutaneous form, as this patient did, a skin biopsy with immunohistochemical staining is diagnostic (Bartlett et al. 2008). Further tests, including blood work, x-rays, and bone marrow specimens may be needed for appropriate staging.

Metastatic carcinoma can resemble anaplastic large cell lymphoma due to the fact that it can display the same type of hallmark cells and growth patterns. The absence of cytokeratin marker militates for anaplastic large cell lymphoma. B-cell lymphoma can be ruled out if the cells test negative for markers of B-cell lineage. These additional tests may be required due to the fact that B-cell lymphomas and rhabdomyosarcomas may test positive for the anaplastic lymphoma kinase protein (Chiarle et al. 2008). However, B-cell non-Hodgkin lymphomas are much less commonly associated with skin involvement than are the T-cell non-Hodgkin lymphomas.

Treatment of anaplastic large cell lymphoma typically involves the use of intensive chemotherapy. Treatment response is often predictable by ALK immunohistochemical staining. ALK-negative anaplastic large cell lymphoma is rarely cured with chemotherapy where ALK positive tumors have a better prognosis. According to a study by Savage et al. on 181 patients, the 5 year overall survival rate for ALK-positive ALCL was approximately 70 %, compared to 49 % for ALK-negative ALCL. However, this study also showed no difference in outcome in patients less than 40 years of age, suggesting that age may be an important prognostic factor in deciding patient outcome (Savage et al. 2008).

New treatments, currently under investigation and review, include medications with anti-CD30 monoclonal antibodies that may be advantageous in destroying ALK-negative tumor cells. Also, ALK-kinase inhibitors may provide a different outlook for treating ALK-positive tumors in the future (Li et al. 2008; McDermott et al. 2008).

Key Points

- Anaplastic large cell lymphoma is a rare form of non-Hodgkin lymphoma (NHL).
- ALK immunohistochemical staining might be helpful in predicting chemotherapeutic response.
- Lymphomas can affect other organs such as the skin, lungs, liver, and bone marrow.

References

Bartlett NL, Younes A, Carabasi MH, Forero A, Rosenblatt JD, Leonard JP, et al. A phase 1 multidose study of SGN-30 immunotherapy in patients with refractory or recurrent CD30+ hematologic malignancies. Blood. 2008;111:1848–54.

Chiarle R, Voena C, Ambrogio C, Piva R, Inghirami G. The anaplastic lymphoma kinase in the pathogenesis of cancer. Nat Rev Cancer. 2008;8:11–23. CrossRefMedlineWeb of Science.

Li R, Morris SW. Development of anaplastic lymphoma kinase (ALK) small-molecule inhibitors for cancer therapy. Med Res Rev. 2008;28:372–412. CrossRefMedlineWeb of Science.

McDermott U, Iafrate AJ, Gray NS, Shioda T, Classon M, Maheswaran S, et al. Genomic alterations of anaplastic lymphoma kinase may sensitize tumors to anaplastic lymphoma kinase inhibitors. Cancer Res. 2008;68:3389–95.

Savage KJ, Harris NL, Vose JM, Ullrich F, Jaffe ES, Connors JM, et al. ALK- anaplastic large-cell lymphoma is clinically and immunophenotypically different from both ALK+ALCL and peripheral T-cell lymphoma, not otherwise specified: report from the International peripheral T-cell lymphoma project. Blood. 2008;111:5496–504.

Stein H, Foss HD, Dürkop H, Marafioti T, Delsol G, Pulford K, et al. CD30(+) Anaplastic large cell lymphoma: a review of its histopathologic, genetic, and clinical features. Blood. 2000;96(12): 3681–95.

Swerdlow SH, Campo E, Harris NL, Jaffe ES, Pileri S, Stein H, et al., editors. WHO classification of tumours of haematopoietic and lymphoid tissues. Lyon: IARC; 2008. p. 312–6.

Chapter 12
Elderly Woman with Large Facial Growth

A 94 year old woman with a history of chronic sun exposure presented with a large, increasingly painful growth (Fig. 12.1). Around 4 months prior to presentation, the patient noticed a pink nodule on the left cheek, which was no larger than a centimeter. For about a month, the size, color and duration of the legion remained constant. One month later, it became darker and rapidly grew to 7 × 8 cm.

Skin biopsy of the left cheek depicted a cellular dermal proliferation of pleomorphic atypical spindle cells with admixed mononuclear cells, multinucleated cells, and foam cells (Fig. 12.1). Immunohistochemical staining showed cells positive for CD10 and CD68, but were negative for S100 and cytokeratin.

Based on the case description, photograph, and histology, what is your diagnosis?

1. Benign fibrous histiocytoma
2. Atypical fibroxanthoma
3. Malignant melanoma
4. Squamous cell carcinoma

R.A. Norman, J. Endo, *Clinical Cases in Geriatric Dermatology,* Clinical Cases in Dermatology, DOI 10.1007/978-1-4471-4135-8_12, © Springer-Verlag London 2013

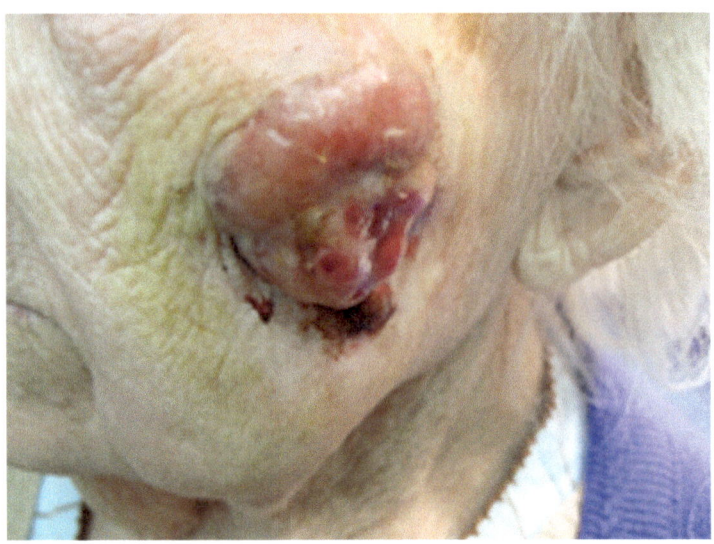

FIGURE 12.1 A 94 year old woman with chronic sun exposure presented with a large facial growth

Diagnosis

Atypical fibroxanthoma

Discussion

Atypical fibroxanthoma, common to elderly patients with years of unprotected sun exposure, frequently appears on the face or the neck (Loo et al. 1993; Rice et al. 1991; Skoulas et al. 2001). It is described as a "low-grade" sarcoma. At first, it appears as a nodule, then it quickly enlarges and ulcerates. Patients typically inquire to a health professional within 4–6 months of its onset. Epidemiologic evidence suggests an increased occurrence in AIDS patients and immunosuppressed transplant patients.

The differential diagnoses for atypical fibroxanthoma are dermatofibrosarcoma protuberans, spindle-cell melanoma, and poorly differentiated squamous cell carcinoma. Immuno-histochemical staining is often required to make the correct diagnosis.

The treatment for atypical fibroxanthoma requires surgical removal. A retrospective case series from Mayo Clinic suggested that Mohs micrographic surgery had lower recurrence rates than wide local excision (Ang 2009). The incidence rate of local reoccurrence is minimal, and metastasis has only been found in exceptional cases.

Key Points

- Atypical fibroxanthomas tend to occur in elderly, chronically sun-exposed patients.
- It is a "low-grade" sarcoma that typically displays a rapid growth phase.
- AIDS or organ transplant patients seem to have a higher risk for developing this sarcoma.

References

Ang GC, Roenigk RK, Otley CC, Kim P, Weaver AL. More than 2 decades of treating atypical fibroxanthoma at mayo clinic: what have we learned from 91 patients? Dermatol Surg. 2009;35(5): 765–72. Epub 2008 Mar 23.

Loo DS, De Pietro WP, Moisa II, Tawfik B. Atypical fibroxanthoma of the cheek: a case report. Cutis. 1993 Jan;51(1):47–8.

Rice CD, Gross DJ, Dinehart SM, Brown HH. Atypical fibroxanthoma of the eyelid and cheek. Arch Ophthalmol. 1991 Jul;109(7):922–3.

Skoulas IG, Price M, Andrew JE, Kountakis SE. Recurrent atypical fibroxanthoma of the cheek. Am J Otolaryngol. 2001;22(1):73–5.

Chapter 13
Purple Mass on Middle Finger

An 81 year old woman with significant sun exposure history presented to our office with a painless purple mass on her middle finger that had rapidly grown over a few months (Fig. 13.1). Upon exam there was an indurated, solitary, 2 cm violaceous nodule.

Based on the case description and the photograph, what is your diagnosis?

1. Squamous cell carcinoma
2. Basal cell carcinoma
3. Melanoma
4. Hemangioma
5. Merkel cell carcinoma

Diagnosis

Merkel cell carcinoma, stage I

R.A. Norman, J. Endo, *Clinical Cases in Geriatric Dermatology,* Clinical Cases in Dermatology, DOI 10.1007/978-1-4471-4135-8_13, © Springer-Verlag London 2013

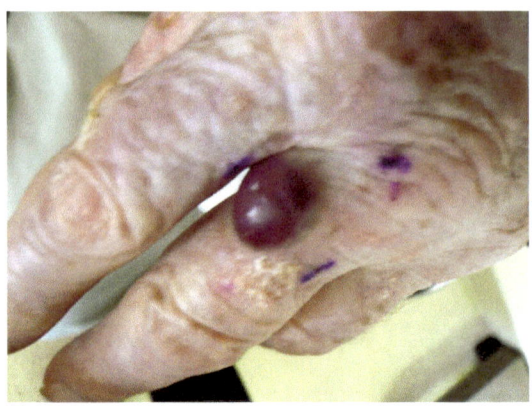

FIGURE 13.1 An 81 year old woman with significant sun exposure history presented with a painless purple mass

Discussion

Merkel cell carcinoma may be associated with a polyoma-virus (Katano et al. 2009). It often appears on sun-exposed areas, such as the head and neck (Calonje 2010 ; Goessling et al. 2006). Clinically, it is often mistaken for a squamous cell carcinoma or cyst. Some studies show men are twice as commonly affected as women. Patients 65 years or older are at a significantly increased risk compared to younger individuals (Albores-Saavedra et al. 2010).

In a recently revised staging system, prognosis is dictated in part by sentinel lymph node status. If it is negative, 5-year-survival rate exceeds 90 %; if positive, survival is 50 % (Gupta 2006). Prognosis might also be based on tumor size, but this remains controversial.

The current treatment algorithm is not based on random-ized control trials due to the fact that the tumor is so rare. Complete excision, whether with Mohs surgery or elliptical excision, is paramount. However, recurrence is still common (Brown et al. 2009). In one study with 5 mm surgical margins, there was 100 % recurrence. Another study showed recurrence of 49 % despite 2.5 cm or greater surgical margins.

Chemotherapy portends higher mortality in some studies. However, the tumor is generally sensitive to radiation therapy.

Key Points

- Merkel cell carcinoma may be associated with a polyomavirus.
- The tumor commonly presents on sun-exposed areas such as the head and neck.
- Merkel cell carcinoma is generally considered a tumor of the elderly or immunocompromised.
- Prognosis is dictated in part by sentinel lymph node status.

References

Albores-Saavedra J, Batich K, Chable-Montero F, Sagy N, Schwartz AM, Henson DE. Merkel cell carcinoma demographics, morphology, and survival based on 3870 cases: a population based study. J Cutan Pathol. 2010;37:20–7.

Brown JA, Smoller BR. Merkel cell carcinoma: what is it, what will it do and where will it go? What role should the pathologist play in reporting this information? J Cutan Pathol. 2009;36:924–7.

Calonje E. Tumours of the skin appendages. In: Burns T, Breathnach S, Cox N, Griffiths C, editors. Rook's textbook of dermatology. 8th ed. Oxford: Wiley-Blackwell; 2010.

Goessling W, Mayer RJ. Merkel cell carcinoma. In: Raghavan D, Brecher ML, Johnson DH, Meropol NJ, Moots PL, Rose PG, Mayer IA, editors. Textbook of uncommon cancer. 3rd ed. Chichester: Wiley; 2006.

Gupta SG, Wang LC, Peñas PF, Gellenthin M, Lee SJ, Nghiem P. Sentinel lymph node biopsy for evaluation and treatment of patients with Merkel cell carcinoma: The Dana-Farber experience and meta-analysis of the literature. Arch Dermatol. 2006 Jun;142(6):685–90.

Katano H, Ito H, Suzuki Y, Nakamura T, Sato Y, Tsuji T, Matsuo K, Nakagawa H, Sata T. Detection of Merkel cell polyomavirus in Merkel cell carcinoma and Kaposi's sarcoma. J Med Virol. 2009;81:1951–8.

Chapter 14
Peeling Rash on the Breast

A 61 year-old female patient presented to the office regarding a 10-month history of a rash on the left breast (Fig. 14.1). There has been progressively more inflammation and itchiness, along with development of surrounding red lesions. There was no history of any trauma to that aspect of the breast. The patient was on previous medications for eczema, but none helped her symptoms.

Based on the case description and the photograph, what is your diagnosis?

1. Mastitis
2. Eczema
3. Contact dermatitis
4. Paget's disease of the breast

Diagnosis

Paget's disease of the breast

R.A. Norman, J. Endo, *Clinical Cases in Geriatric Dermatology,* Clinical Cases in Dermatology, DOI 10.1007/978-1-4471-4135-8_14, © Springer-Verlag London 2013

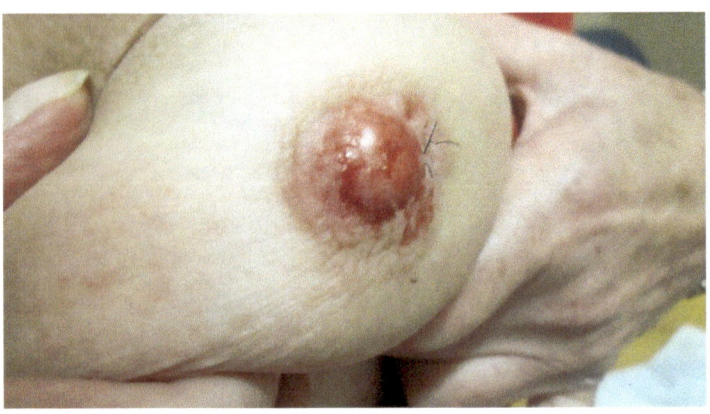

FIGURE 14.1 A 61 year-old female patient presented for evaluation of a rash that was located on the left breast

Discussion

Mammary Paget's disease is a malignant disease that is often confused with eczema, due to the scaling and crusting on and around the nipple. Studies have shown that mammary Paget's disease with or without a palpable mass associated with changes in the nipple, correlates with an underlying breast carcinoma in at least 95 % of cases. The incidence of mammary Paget's disease is almost completely confined to the female population. The mean age of diagnosis for female patients is approximately 55 years (Valdes 2006).

Extramammary Paget's is a related condition that involves can involve other anatomic sites in both genders. Although the histological aspects of both of these conditions are alike, there is likely a different pathophysiology.

To help aid in the diagnosis, it is recommended that females suspected of having Paget's disease of the nipple undergo mammogram and biopsy. Cytopathology may also aid in further analysis.

The treatment of choice is tumor excision and lymph node dissection. However, the surgical approach is related to whether there is a palpable underlying breast mass. In those with a palpable mass, a modified radical is often recommended. If a palpable tumor is not present, a more conservative resection, with or without radiation therapy, is suggested. The overall survival rate for these patients is significantly higher for the latter group (Dalberg et al. 2008).

Key Points

- Mammary Paget's disease is a cutaneous adenocarcinoma that is often associated with an underlying breast cancer.
- Most patients with mammary Paget's disease are older females.
- The usual presentation is "refractory eczema" that often affects the nipple.

References

Dalberg K, Hellborg H, Wärnberg F. Paget's disease of the nipple in a population based cohort. Breast Cancer Res Treat. 2008; 111(2):313–9.

Valdes EK, Feldman SM. Paget's disease of the breast. Breast J. 2006; 12(1):83.

Chapter 15
A 67 Year Old Female with Scaly Plaques

A 67 year-old female presented with erythematous and pruritic diffuse scaly plaques on the upper back, arms, and neck for 4 years (Figs. 15.1, 15.2, and 15.3). Over the last year the arm lesions had become thickened, hyperkeratotic, and demarcated. She had used over the counter cortisone cream that provided minimal relief. A potassium hydroxide (KOH) skin scraping was negative. A biopsy was performed.

Based on the case description and the photograph, what is your diagnosis?

1. Tinea
2. Psoriasis
3. Subacute dermatitis
4. Mycosis fungoides

Diagnosis

Mycosis fungoides

R.A. Norman, J. Endo, *Clinical Cases in Geriatric Dermatology,* Clinical Cases in Dermatology, DOI 10.1007/978-1-4471-4135-8_15, © Springer-Verlag London 2013

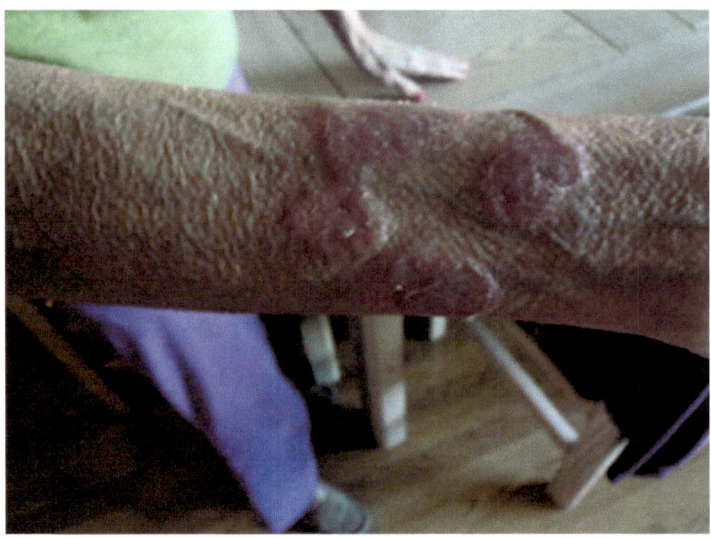

Figure 15.1 A 67 year-old female presented with erythematous and pruritic diffuse scaly plaques on the arms, upper back, and neck for 4 years

Discussion

Mycosis fungoides (MF) is the most common primary cutaneous T-cell lymphoma (CTCL). Its name is somewhat of a misnomer; the condition is not actually fungal infection but rather a primary cutaneous form of non-Hodgkin lymphoma. The age of onset is the fifth decade of life (Cerroni et al. 2005). It is twice as common in men as in women. The pathogenesis is unknown.

Lesions in early stages appear in patches, and are erythematous and pruritic. The lesions tend to favor unexposed areas of the skin (under breasts, buttocks, lower abdomen, groin). Eventually the patchy lesions can become thickened. In the plaque stage, hyperkeratotic, demarcated and appear as psoriasiform plaques (James et al. 2006). In the tumor stage, nodules arise from the plaques and can become painful

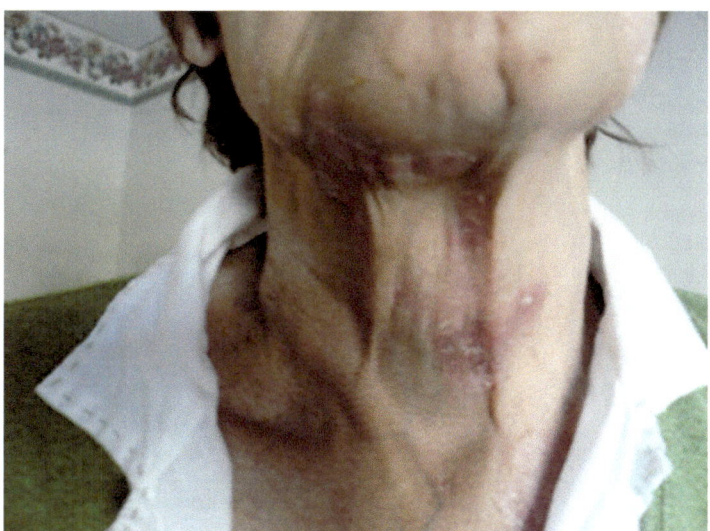

FIGURE 15.2 A 67 year-old female presented with erythematous and pruritic diffuse scaly plaques on the neck

and ulcerated. These lesions are most commonly found on the trunk. The erythrodermic stage manifests as large areas of erythema, lymphadenopathy, and circulating abnormal Sezary cells. Nails and hair can be involved.

The worst prognosis of MF is associated with >10 % skin involvement, presence of tumors, lymphadenopathy, and generalized erythroderma (Zackheim 1999).

The diagnosis of early stage MF often requires multiple biopsies even with a skilled dermatopathologist. Histologic confirmation of MF may not be achieved for many years. If the biopsied lesion has a CD8+ T cell component of more than 20 % involvement, a correlation can be made with a better prognosis for the patient (Lenane et al. 2007).

Treatment can induce remission, but no clear therapy has been proven to prolong survival. Quality of life in conjunction with extending remission are the primary treatment goals. Treatment for MF typically varies depending on the stage of involvement and the location of the lesions (James 2006).

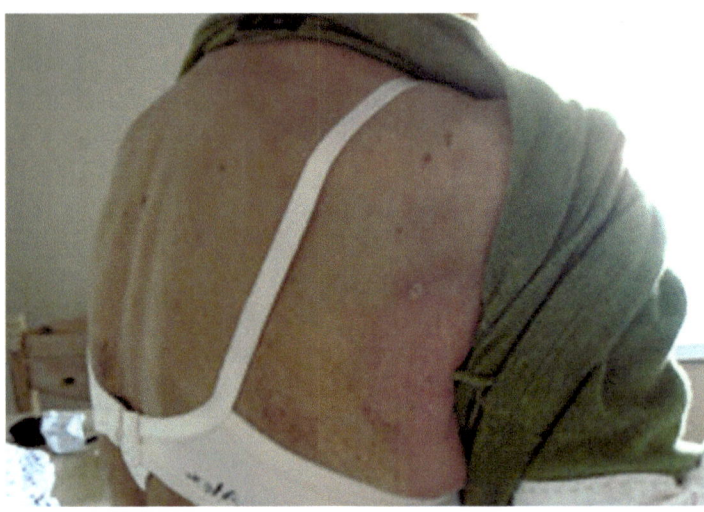

FIGURE 15.3 A 67 year-old female presented with erythematous and pruritic diffuse scaly patches on the upper back

PUVA, topical chemotherapy (such as nitrogen mustard), and ultrapotent corticosteroids are the most effective treatments for early stages of the disease. Oral or topical retinoids, electron beam therapy, systemic chemotherapy, interferon-alpha, newer targeted immunotherapies, and extracorporeal photophoresis have been used in more advanced stages of the disease. In 2010, the FDA approved a naloxone lotion, which acts by way of antagonizing opioid receptors that can be utilized as treatment for the pruritus associated with cutaneous T-cell lymphoma (Wolff et al. 2005).

Key Points

- Mycosis fungoides (MF) is the most common type of cutaneous T-cell lymphoma (CTCL), which is a family of primary cutaneous non-Hodgkin's lymphoma.
- The age of onset is the fifth decade of life, and more than women are affected.

- Early stage can mimic "refractory" eczema, and multiple biopsies, even with a skilled dermatopathologist, are sometimes required to clinch the diagnosis.

References

Cerroni L, Gatter K, Kerl H. An illustrated guide to skin lymphomas. Malden: Blackwell Publishing; 2005. p. 13.

James WD, Berger TG, Elston DM. Andrews' diseases of the skin clinical dermatology. 10th ed. Philadelphia: Saunders, Elsevier; 2006. p. 727–33.

Lenane P, Powell FC, O'Keane C, et al. Mycosis fungoides-a review of the management of 28 patients and of the recent literature. Int Soc of Dermatol. 2007;46:19–26.

Wolff K, Dick S, Johnson RA. Fitzpatrick's color atlas & synopsis of clinical dermatology. 5th ed. New York: McGraw-Hill; 2005. p. 528–31.

Zackheim HS, Amin S, Kashani-Sabet M, McMillan A. Prognosis in cutaneous T-cell lymphoma by skin stage: Long-term survival in 489 patients. J Am Acad Dermatol. 1999;40(3):418–25.

Chapter 16
Slow Growing Lesion on the Top of Head

A 75 year old man presented with a slow-growing lesion usually on the top of his head (Fig. 16.1). He explained that the lesion bled and has recurred after he tried to scrape it off.

Based on the case description and the photograph, what is your diagnosis?

1. Squamous cell carcinoma
2. Basal cell carcinoma
3. Melanoma
4. Melanocytic nevus
5. Seborrheic keratosis

Diagnosis

Basal cell carcinoma

Discussion

Basal cell carcinomas can take on a wide variety of manifestations, including nodular (pearly, translucent with telangiectasias), pigmented (spots of gray and blue), morpheaform

R.A. Norman, J. Endo, *Clinical Cases in Geriatric Dermatology,* Clinical Cases in Dermatology, DOI 10.1007/978-1-4471-4135-8_16, © Springer-Verlag London 2013

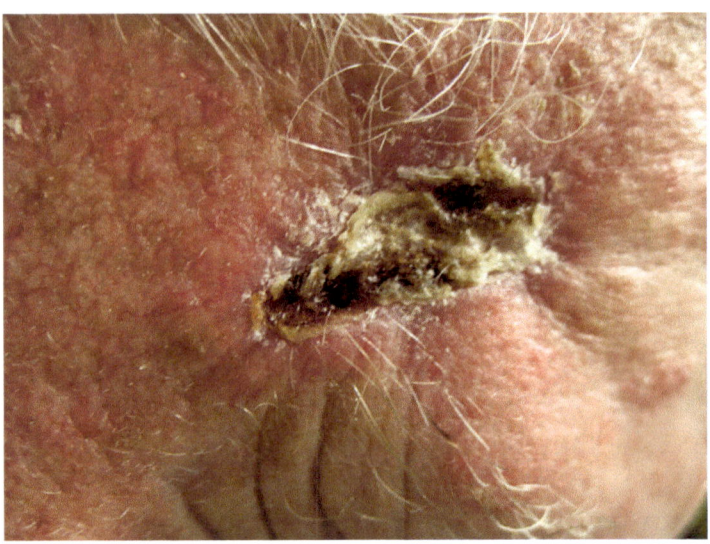

FIGURE 16.1 An 75 year old man presented with a slow-growing lesion on his head

(poorly demarcated and scar-like), and superficial (pink to brown and sometimes eczematous appearance) (Freedberg et al. 2003; James et al. 2006).

Depending upon anatomic site, size, histologic features, and patient preference, therapy can include:

- Destruction by electrodesiccation & curettage
- Cryotherapy
- Elliptical excision
- Topical therapy with 5-fluorouracil or imiquimod for superficial variants
- Orthovoltage radiation therapy for non-surgical candidates
- Mohs micrographic surgery in recurrent cases, immuno-suppressed patients, cosmetically sensitive anatomic sites, histologically aggressive variants, or "high-risk" sites of recurrence such as the "H-zone" of the face (Maloney et al. 1999 ; Wolf et al. 1987). The American Academy of Dermatology has published the 2012 Mohs Appropriate

Use Guidelines. It is available at http://www.aad.org/education-and-quality-care/appropriate-use-criteria/mohs-surgery-auc.

Key Points

- Basal cell carcinoma is the most common skin cancer and is related to sun exposure.
- The classic nodular variant has pearliness and telangiectasias, but the astute practitioner must be aware of the other variants that can mimic scars, eczema, and pigmented lesions.
- Treatment depends upon multiple patient and tumor histologic factors.
- The American Academy of Dermatology has published appropriate use guidelines for Mohs surgery.

References

Freedberg IM, Freedberg IM, et al. Fitzpatrick's dermatology in general medicine. 6th ed. New York: McGraw-Hill; 2003.

James WD, Berger TG, et al. Andrews' diseases of the skin: clinical dermatology. Philadelphia: Saunders Elsevier; 2006.

Maloney ME, et al. Surgical dermatopathology. Cambridge: Blackwell; 1999. p. 110.

Wolf DJ, Zitelli JA. Surgical margins for basal cell carcinoma. Arch Dermatol. 1987;123(3):340–4.

Chapter 17
71 Year Old Woman with Itchy Rash on Breast

A 68-year-old woman had a 2-month history of a pruritic eruption on the right breast. Six months earlier, she underwent a mastectomy for breast cancer and had a tissue expander placed in anticipation of a breast reconstruction procedure. She had applied an antifungal cream without improvement of the rash.

On examination, there is a red, poorly defined, nonsubstantive plaque on the breast, with fine scale and crust on the surface (Fig. 17.1). There is no palpable regional lymphadenopathy. The right breast is not involved.

Based on the case description and the photograph, what is your diagnosis?

1. Contact dermatitis
2. Pressure necrosis
3. Resistant tinea corporis
4. Impetigo
5. Breast metastasis

Diagnosis

Breast metastasis

R.A. Norman, J. Endo, *Clinical Cases in Geriatric Dermatology,* Clinical Cases in Dermatology, DOI 10.1007/978-1-4471-4135-8_17, © Springer-Verlag London 2013

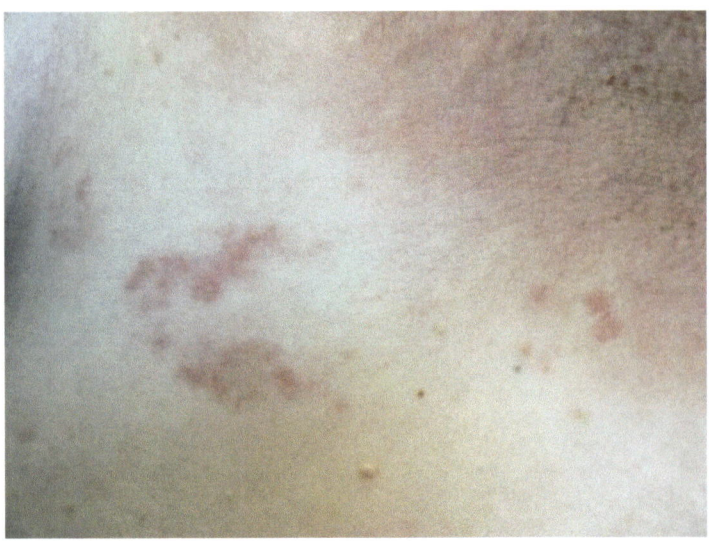

FIGURE 17.1 A red, poorly defined, nonsubstantive plaque on the breast, with fine scale and crust on the surface

Discussion

Breast carcinoma can spread to overlying skin through regional lymphatics (De Giorgi et al. 2010; Fisher et al. 1975; Hussein 2010) but can also metastasize to distant sites such as the scalp. Contrary to other cutaneous metastatic diseases, breast cancer metastases are not always palpable papules or nodules but can manifest as inflammatory red patches or minimally scaly or crusted plaques on the chest wall (Krathen et al. 2003; Nashan et al. 2010; Schwartz 2008).

Our patient was referred back to her oncologist for consideration of further surgery and chemotherapy.

Contact dermatitis from topical medication or some other allergen can cause a red, itchy, crusted, nonsubstantive plaque. One would expect more surface change (weeping, oozing, crusting, and blistering) with this condition.

Pressure necrosis of the skin overlying the tissue expander could cause crusting, but the lack of a necrotic eschar fails to support this diagnosis.

Tinea corporis can cause a unilateral, scaly, erythematous plaque, similar to what is seen in this case. However, the scale is typically at the advancing margin of the lesion rather than in the center. Potassium hydroxide preparation of skin scraping can be a fast, inexpensive test. Given the patient's history, lack of response to topical antifungals, cutaneous metastasis should be ruled out with skin biopsy.

Impetigo commonly causes a yellow-crusted, localized, inflamed plaque. The relatively small amount of surface change as compared with the amount of erythema makes this less likely.

Key Point

- Patients with a personal or strong family history of breast cancer presenting with asymmetric patches, papules, plaques, or nodules on the chest wall should have a skin biopsy to exclude cutaneous adenocarcinoma metastasis.

References

De Giorgi V, Grazzini M, Alfaioli B, Savarese I, Corciova SA, Guerriero G, Lotti T. Cutaneous manifestations of breast carcinoma. Dermatol Ther. 2010;23:581–9.

Fisher ER, Gregorio RM, Fisher B, With the Assistance of Carol Redmond ScD, Vellios F, Sommers SC, Cooperating Investigators. The pathology of invasive breast cancer A Syllabus Derived from Findings of the National Surgical Adjuvant Breast Project (Protocol No. 4). Cancer. 1975;36:1–85.

Hussein MRA. Skin metastasis: a pathologist's perspective. J Cutan Pathol. 2010;37:e1–20.

Krathen RA, Orengc IF, Rosen T. Cutaneous metastasis: a meta-analysis of data. South Med J. 2003;96(2):164–7.

Nashan D, Meiss F, Braun-Falco M, Reichenberger S. Cutaneous metastases from internal malignancies. Dermatol Ther. 2010;23:567–80.

Schwartz RA. Cutaneous metastatic disease, in skin cancer: recognition and management. 2nd ed. Oxford: Blackwell; 2008.

Chapter 18
82 Year Old with Pigmented Lesion

An 82-year-old female patient presented with a dark and irregular lesion in an area of chronically sun exposed skin (Fig. 18.1). She had no previous treatment. A biopsy was performed.

Based on the case description and the photograph, what is your diagnosis?

1. Solar lentigo
2. Fixed drug eruption
3. Lentigo maligna
4. Post-inflammatory hyperpigmentation
5. Pigmented basal cell carcinoma

Diagnosis

Lentigo maligna

Discussion

Lentigo maligna is melanoma in-situ that occurs in chronically sun-exposed skin of the elderly. Typically this presents as darkening, changing borders or colors within a preexisting

R.A. Norman, J. Endo, *Clinical Cases in Geriatric Dermatology,* Clinical Cases in Dermatology, DOI 10.1007/978-1-4471-4135-8_18, © Springer-Verlag London 2013

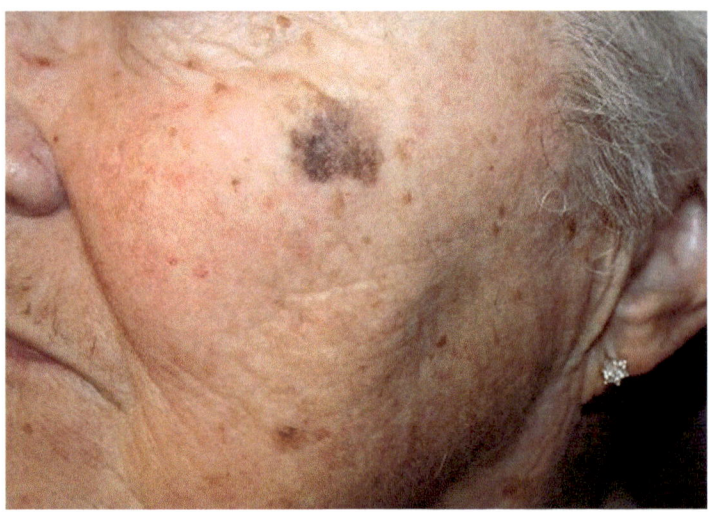

Figure 18.1 The patient showed a dark and irregular lesion in an area of chronically sun exposed skin

lentigo (sun spot) (James et al. 2006; Stevenson et al. 2005; Weinstock et al. 1987).

The overall incidence of cutaneous melanoma is increasing faster than that of any other neoplasm (Bub et al. 2004; Hazan et al. 2008; McKenna et al. 2006). Lentigo maligna (LM) represents 5–15 % of melanoma cases and is generally considered a slow-growing variant. It is thought that less than 5 % progress to have an invasive component, which is called lentigo maligna melanoma (LMM) (Bolognia 2008). Treatment for lentigo maligna is somewhat controversial and evolving. Options include Mohs surgery, radiotherapy, and topical imiquimod (Bolognia 2008; Hyde 2012).

Solar lentigo appears in areas of sun damage, as in this case. However, they are usually smaller and have more uniform color and borders.

Fixed drug eruption is a circular, often hyperpigmented patch that intermittent appears in the same location after recurrent exposures to the ingestant.

Post-inflammatory hyperpigmentation can occur on the face as a linear brown patch on the face. However, the irregularity of the margins of the lesion and the lack of a history of a preceding inflammatory process makes this diagnosis less likely.

Pigmented basal cell carcinoma usually appears as a firm lesion that is raised, shiny, and pearly, and the area may bleed following minor injury. Although basal cell carcinoma is often pink or red, the pigmented variant can appear similar to a melanoma.

Key Points

- Lentigo maligna is melanoma in situ on chronically sun-damaged skin of older patients.
- A minority of lentigo maligna (LM) lesions slowly progress to invasive lentigo maligna melanoma (LMM).

References

Bolognia J, Jorizzo JL, Rapini RP. Dermatology. St. Louis: Mosby/Elsevier; 2008.

Bub JL, Berg D, Slee A, Odland PB. Management of lentigo maligna and lentigo maligna melanoma with staged excision: a 5-year follow-up. Arch Dermatol. 2004;140(5):552–8.

Hazan C, Dusza SW, Delgado R, Busam KJ, Halpern AC, Nehal KS. Staged excision for lentigo maligna and lentigo maligna melanoma: a retrospective analysis of 117 cases. J Am Acad Dermatol. 2008; 58(1):142–8.

Hyde MA, Hadley ML, Tristani-Firouzi P, Goldgar D, Bowen GM. A randomized trial of the off-label use of imiquimod, 5%, cream with vs without tazarotene, 0.1%, gel for the treatment of lentigo maligna, followed by conservative staged excisions. Arch Dermatol. 2012;148(5):592–6.

James William D, Berger Timothy G, et al. Andrews' diseases of the skin: clinical dermatology. Philadelphia: Saunders Elsevier; 2006.

McKenna JK, Florell SR, Goldman GD, Bowen GM. Lentigo maligna/lentigo maligna melanoma: current state of diagnosis and treatment. Dermatol Surg. 2006;32(4):493–504.

Stevenson O, Ahmed I. Lentigo maligna: prognosis and treatment options. Am J Clin Dermatol. 2005;6(3):151–64.

Weinstock MA, Sober AJ. The risk of progression of lentigo maligna to lentigo maligna melanoma. Br J Dermatol. 1987;116(3):303–10.

Chapter 19
Scaly Lesion on the Lip

A 63 year old man presented with a scaly and ulcerated nodule on his lower lip (Fig. 19.1). He had a history of being
outside without using sunscreen.

   Based on the case description and the photograph, what is
your diagnosis?

1. Squamous cell carcinoma
2. Basal cell carcinoma
3. Melanoma
4. Melanocytic nevus
5. Actinic keratosis

Diagnosis

Squamous cell carcinoma

Discussion

Squamous cell carcinoma (SCC) is a malignancy of keratinocytes with full-thickness atypia of the epidermis. It is thought
to arise from actinic keratoses, which are "pre-cancerous" pink,

R.A. Norman, J. Endo, *Clinical Cases in Geriatric*   85
Dermatology, Clinical Cases in Dermatology,
DOI 10.1007/978-1-4471-4135-8_19,
© Springer-Verlag London 2013

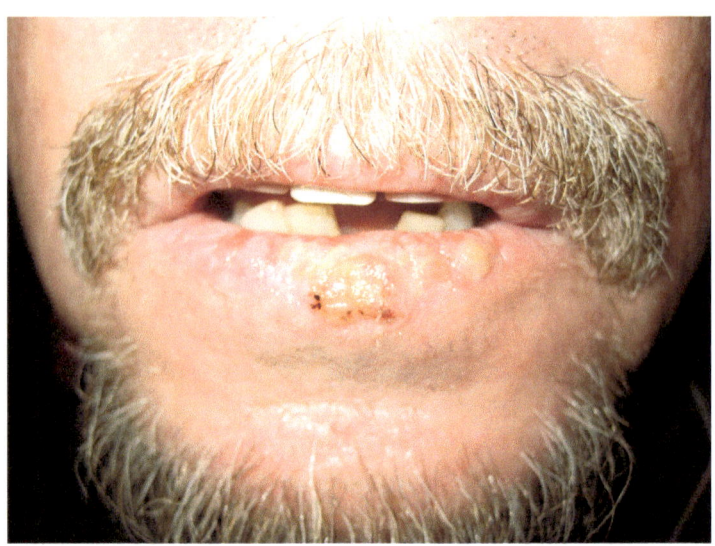

FIGURE 19.1   A 63 year old man presented with a scaly and ulcerated lesion on his lower lip

rough, scaly papules that exhibit partial thickness keratinocyte atypia. SCC commonly occurs in sun-exposed skin areas, including the lips, ears, upper extremities, and face. The appearance of squamous cell carcinoma can be highly variable. Typically, the tumor is an ulcerated or scaly red plaque or nodule that grows slowly. It can also display raised edges around the ulceration (Schwartz 2008; Scully 2008; Veness 2005).

In addition to chronic sun damage, chronic immunosuppression is another major risk factor. For this reason, solid organ transplant patients are recommended to have annual skin cancer screening (Kasiske et al., 2000).

Diagnosis is typically done with a incisional or punch biopsy or shave biopsy with adequate depth. Histologic prognostic feature include tumor depth, degree of invasion and atypia, and the presence of perineural invasion. The Seventh Edition of the American Joint Committee on Cancer (AJCC) guidelines now recommend Breslow depth reporting similar to melanoma, although this has not been widely adapted yet at the time of this writing (Warner 2011).

Treatment includes simple excision, Mohs micrographic surgery, electrodessication & curettage, and Aldara (imiquimod) based upon anatomic site, tumor size & histologic features, and patient preference (Bolognia 2008; Bonerandi et al. 2011; Quinn et al. 2010).

References

Bolognia J, Jorizzo JL, Rapini RP. Dermatology. St. Louis: Mosby/Elsevier; 2008.

Bonerandi J, Beauvillain C, Caquant L, Chassagne J, Chaussade V, Clavère P, Desouches C, Garnier F, Grolleau J, Grossin M, Jourdain A, Lemonnier J, Maillard H, Ortonne N, Rio E, Simon E, Sei J, Grob J, Martin L, French Dermatology Recommendations Association (aRED). Guidelines for the diagnosis and treatment of cutaneous squamous cell carcinoma and precursor lesions. J Eur Acad Dermatol Venereol. 2011;25:1–51.

Kasiske BL, Vazquez MA, Harmon WE, Brown RS, Danovitch GM, Gaston RS, Roth D, Scandling JD, Singer GG. Recommendations for the outpatient surveillance of renal transplant recipients. American Society of Transplantation. J Am Soc Nephrol. 2000 Oct;11 Suppl 15:S1–86.

Quinn AG, Perkins W. Non-melanoma skin cancer and other epidermal skin tumours. In: Burns T, Breathnach S, Cox N, Griffiths C, editors. Rook's textbook of dermatology. 8th ed. Oxford: Wiley-Blackwell; 2010.

Schwartz RA. Squamous cell carcinoma. In: Skin cancer: recognition and management. 2nd ed. Oxford: Blackwell; 2008.

Scully C. The oral cavity and lips. In: Burns T, Breathnach S, Cox N, Griffiths C, editors. Rook's textbook of dermatology. 7th ed. Malden: Blackwell; 2008.

Veness M. Treatment recommendations in patients diagnosed with high-risk cutaneous squamous cell carcinoma. Australas Radiol. 2005;49:365–76.

Warner C, Cockerell C. The new seventh edition American Joint Committee on cancer staging of cutaneous non-melanoma skin cancer: a critical review. Am J Clin Dermatol. 2011;12(3):147–54.

Chapter 20
Painful Mass on Ring Finger

A 51 year-old male presented to the office complaining of an 8-month history of a 3 cm, steadily growing mass on his left ring finger, along the distal interphalangeal joint (Fig. 20.1). He also was experiencing worsening pain, and the mass had once oozed liquid. There was no history of any trauma. The patient was not on any medications and denied any past treatments for this condition.

Based on the case description and the photograph, what is your diagnosis?

1. Foreign body granuloma
2. Giant cell tumor of tendon sheath
3. Rheumatoid nodule
4. Synovial chondromatosis
5. Periosteal chondroma
6. Myxoid cyst

A skin biopsy demonstrated giant cells encapsulated within collagen.

R.A. Norman, J. Endo, *Clinical Cases in Geriatric Dermatology,* Clinical Cases in Dermatology, DOI 10.1007/978-1-4471-4135-8_20, © Springer-Verlag London 2013

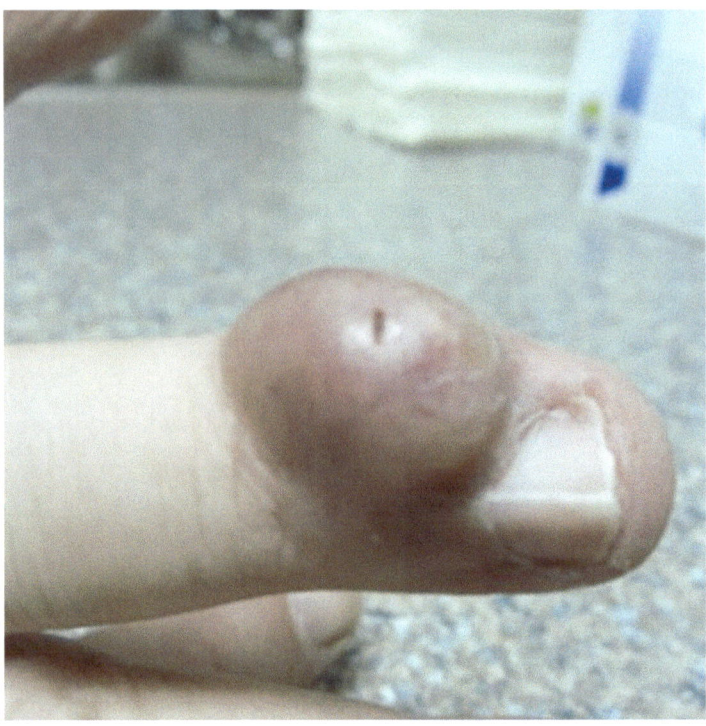

FIGURE 20.1 A 51 year-old male presented to the office complaining of an 8-month history of a 3 cm, steadily growing mass on his left ring finger along the distal interphalangeal joint

Diagnosis

Giant cell tumor of tendon sheath

Discussion

Giant cell tumor of the tendon sheath is the second most common tumor of the hand after ganglion cysts. The etiology is currently unknown. Its texture is rubbery and the color can range from gray, to yellow, to orange (Abdul-Karim et al. 1992;

Abimelec et al. 1996). Histologically, the tumor cells are infiltrated with a mixture of synovial cells, multinucleated giant cells, macrophages, and xanthoma cells.

Giant cell tumors of tendon sheath typically occur in males. These tumors can be categorized into two different types: localized and diffuse. The localized form is most common and usually affects the upper extremities, with a preference for the flexor surface of both the hand and wrist (Jones et al. 1969). The rare diffuse form is related to diffuse pigmented villonodular synovitis (PVNS) and has a predilection for the lower extremities, most frequently around the patella. PVNS is more aggressive clinically, and tends to recur even after surgical removal (Murphey et al. 2008).

This is a diagnosis by biopsy. Plain radiographs are beneficial in half of cases and may demonstrate cortical erosion of the underlying bone, especially if the tumor is particularly painful.

The treatment of choice for a giant cell tumor of tendon sheath is careful surgical excision, although recurrences can occur between 9–44% of the time. Piercing the lesion should be avoided as the tumor cells may spread to neighboring tissues.

References

Abdul-Karim FW, el-Naggar AK, Joyce MJ. Diffuse and localized tenosynovial giant cell tumor and pigmented villonodular synovitis: a clinicopathologic and flow cytometric DNA analysis. Hum Pathol. 1992;23(7):729–35.

Abimelec P, Cambiaghi S, Thioly D. Subungual giant cell tumor of the tendon sheath. Cutis. 1996;58(4):273–5.

Jones FE, Soule EH, Coventry MB. Fibrous xanthoma of synovium (giant-cell tumor of tendon sheath, pigmented nodular synovitis). A study of one hundred and eighteen cases. J Bone Joint Surg Am. 1969;51(1):76–86.

Murphey MD, Rhee JH, Lewis RB, Fanburg-Smith JC, Flemming DJ, Walker EA. Pigmented villonodular synovitis: radiologic-pathologic correlation. Radiographics. 2008;28(5):1493–518.

Part IV
Inflammatory Disorders

Chapter 21
A 66 Year Old Woman with a Blistering Eruption

66-year-old woman with a 1 week history of a itchy and blistering eruption of the hands. The lesions started as very pruritic, small vesicles that subsequently spread to involve her palms and backs of her hands (Fig. 21.1). She relates this to working in her garden without gloves. She reports no recent history of a similar outbreak.

On examination, there is marked bilateral erythema, edema, and vesiculation, with pustules on the fingers as well as the palmar and dorsal hands.

Based on the case description and the photograph, what is your diagnosis?

1. Bullous pemphigoid
2. Tinea manuum
3. Contact dermatitis

Diagnosis

Contact dermatitis

R.A. Norman, J. Endo, *Clinical Cases in Geriatric Dermatology,* Clinical Cases in Dermatology, DOI 10.1007/978-1-4471-4135-8_21, © Springer-Verlag London 2013

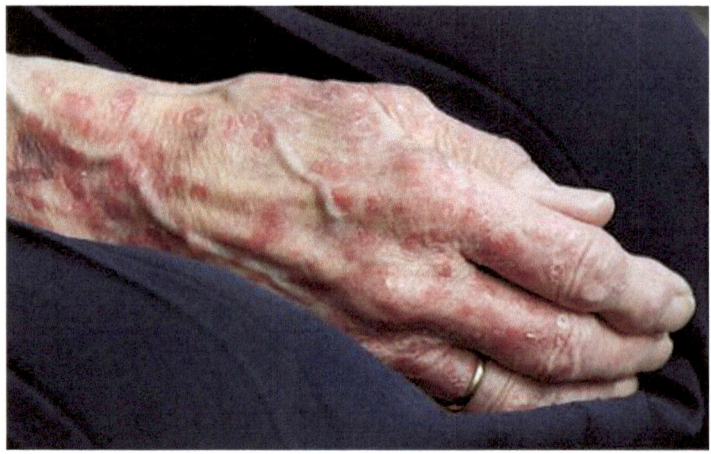

FIGURE 21.1 A 66-year-old woman with a 1 week history of a itchy and blistering eruption of the hands

Discussion

Contact dermatitis has classically been divided into allergic and irritant causes. Allergic causes (e.g., poison ivy dermatitis) require sensitization to the antigen and subsequent re-exposure. Allergic contact dermatitis is a delayed type IV reaction, with a classic 2 day window between re-exposure and symptom onset. The areas of demarcation are often well-defined. Irritant dermatitis (e.g., bleach exposure), in contradistinction, does not require sensitization (Bourke et al. 2001; Beck et al. 2010; Cohen et al. 1997; Elsner et al. 1990). Sometimes the vesiculation or pustules is mistaken for a primary infectious etiology. However, it is important to highlight that an acute and exuberant contact dermatitis can cause the degree of vesiculation (dyshidrosis) and pustules noted in this case (Kimber et al. 2002; Morris-Jones et al. 2002; Wilkinson et al. 2008).

Topical preparations containing ingredients such as vitamin E, fragrances, parabens, diphenhydramine (Benadryl spray, Caladryl lotion), neomycin (Neosporin), and PABA (paraamino benzoic acid) are common allergenic offenders. Overuse of bar soaps, harsh cleansers, alcohol-containing moisturizers, and cosmetics can produce irritation. An important clinical pearl is patients with stasis dermatitis seem to be at higher risk for developing contact dermatitis (Prakash 2010).

Diagnosis

Generally a good history and skin examination are sufficient to diagnosis dermatitis. Skin scraping with potassium hydroxide (KOH) mounting can be considered in some cases to exclude dermatophytosis (tinea manuum) or scabies. Biopsy is sometimes considered if other causes, particularly psoriasis, are suspected. Patch testing can be helpful if patients do not respond to topical steroids or those whose history and occupation suggest a likely allergic contact dermatitis.

Therapy

1. Discontinue offending allergic topical agents
2. Mild or midstrength steroids are preferable to high potency topical steroids in the elderly to avoid atrophy
3. Apply soothing, cool compresses, followed by bland emollients to reduce itch.

Pustular psoriasis may be a recurrent process, but typically produces pustules rather than vesicles of the hands. Family history and examination findings of psoriasiform lesions of the nails or elsewhere on the skin can be helpful.

Tinea manuum (fungal infection of the hands) can produce vesicles. The degree of inflammation with the very significant edema observed in our case would be atypical for dermatophytosis. Potassium hydroxide scraping can be helpful to look for the dermotophytes.

Bullous pemphigoid rarely develops on the palms alone, at least initially. A skin biopsy with immunofluorescent studies would be needed to confirm the diagnosis.

Key Points

- Contact dermatitis occurs in the elderly, especially those with comorbid stasis dermatitis.
- A careful history (including all over-the-counter medicaments) and physical exam clues can suggest potential causes of allergic contact dermatitis.
- When patients do not respond to topical steroids and emollients, skin biopsy and/or patch testing can be considered.

References

Bourke J, Coulson I, English J. Guidelines for care of contact dermatitis. Br J Dermatol. 2001;145(6):877–85.

Beck MH, Wilkinson SM. Contact dermatitis: allergic. In: Burns T, Breathnach S, Cox N, Griffiths C, editors. Rook's textbook of dermatology. 8th ed. Oxford: Wiley-Blackwell; 2010.

Cohen DE, Brancaccio R, Andersen D, Belsito DV. Utility of a standard allergen series alone in the evaluation of allergic contact dermatitis: a retrospective study of 732 patients. J Am Acad Dermatol. 1997; 36(6 Pt 1):914–8.

Elsner P, Wilhelm D, Maibach HI. Irritant contact dermatitis irritant contact dermatitis and aging. Contact Dermatitis. 1990;23:275.

Kimber I, Basketter DA, Gerberick GF, Dearman RJ. Allergic contact dermatitis. Int Immunopharmacol. 2002;2(2–3):201–11.

Morris-Jones R, Robertson SJ, Ross JS, White IR, McFadden JP, Rycroft RJ. Dermatitis caused by physical irritants. Br J Dermatol. 2002;147(2):270–5.

Prakash AV, Davis MD. Contact dermatitis in older adults: a review of the literature. Am J Clin Dermatol. 2010;11(6):373–81.

Wilkinson SM, Beck MH. Contact dermatitis: irritant. In: Burns T, Breathnach S, Cox N, Griffiths C, editors. Rook's textbook of dermatology. 7th ed. Malden: Blackwell Publishing, Inc.; 2008.

Chapter 22
71 Year Old Man with Dry Skin

A 71 year old male complained of chronically dry skin on his lower extremities that has progressed over the last year (Fig. 22.1). Over the counter moisturizers help, but it has not stopped the dryness and the itching.

Based on the case description and the photograph, what is your diagnosis?

1. Numular dermatitis
2. Xerosis
3. Stasis dermatitis
4. Ichthyosis vulgaris

Diagnosis

Xerosis (winter itch, asteatotic dermatitis)

Discussion

Xerotic skin appears dry, rough and scaly due to moisture loss from the stratum corneum. In severe cases, marked fissuring can lead to a "crazy pavement" appearance (eczema craquele) (Judge et al. 2010; Norman 2003; Proksch et al. 2005; Rapini et al. 2007). Pruritus is often present and may be

R.A. Norman, J. Endo, *Clinical Cases in Geriatric Dermatology,* Clinical Cases in Dermatology, DOI 10.1007/978-1-4471-4135-8_22, © Springer-Verlag London 2013

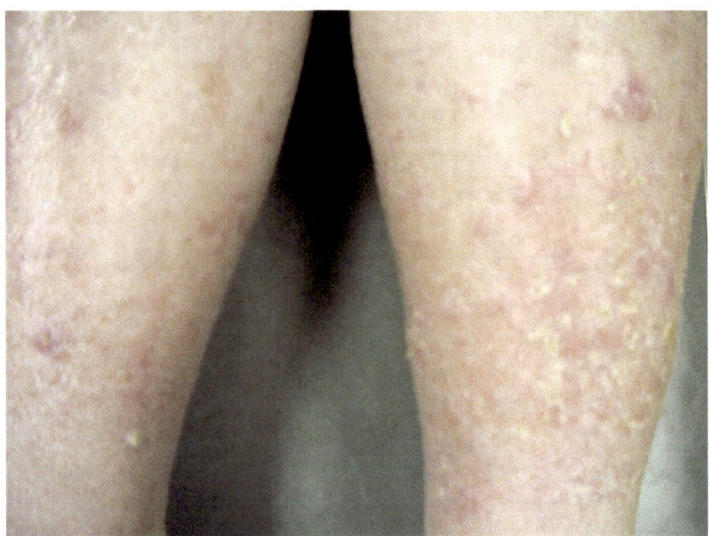

FIGURE 22.1 A 71 year old male complained of chronically dry skin on his lower extremities that has progressed over the last year

localized or generalized. The condition is aggravated during the winter months by low humidity, cold and windy weather, dry heat, and excessive bathing.

Although xerosis may be triggered by drugs or physical health problems, it is usually not associated with a systemic disease. Nonetheless, a history of preexisting diseases, conditions, therapies, and medications may contribute to making the elderly more susceptible to xerosis. Such a history may include prior irradiation, advanced renal disease, zinc or essential fatty acid deficiencies, thyroid disease, diuretic therapy, human immunodeficiency virus (HIV) and malignancies (Norman 2003). Generally, a biopsy is not needed to make this clinical diagnosis.

Differential Diagnosis

1. Nummular dermatitis shows discrete, red, annular, scaly, dry patches on the arms and legs.

2. Ichthyosis vulgaris is an autosomal dominant disorder, often associated with atopic dermatitis, hyperlinear palms, and keratosis pilaris (keratotic, 1–2-mm red-brown follicular papules on the upper outer arms and anterior thighs).
3. Stasis dermatitis is an itchy, red rash of the lower extremities that is usually associated with venous insufficiency. There can be a brown hue from hemosiderin deposition under the skin.

Treatment

1. Artificial humidification with a home humidifier
2. Less frequent bathing, using warm rather than hot water, and focusing on visibly soiled skin and intertriginous areas.
3. The use of a mild soap or cleansing cream (e.g., Dove soap, Cetaphil, Cerave) rather than harsh, antibacterial, or bar soaps.
4. The patient should wear protective clothing in cold weather.
5. Occlusive moisturizers (e.g., petrolatum) coat the surface of the skin, reducing the evaporative loss of moisture from the surface (Schafer-Korting et al. 1989; Van Scott et al. 1974 ; Wehr et al. 1986).

The use of bath oils for bathing can be extremely hazardous for the elderly because of the increased possibility of slipping in the tub. Creams and moisturizers should be applied after getting out of the bathtub or shower. At that time, the body should be patted with a towel and the moisturizing preparation applied within a few minutes. Under these conditions, the skin is fully hydrated and the moisturizing preparation is more effective in preventing epidermal water loss.

Humectant moisturizers containing urea and lactic acid may not be tolerated because of irritation but are very effective in improving keratinocyte moisture retention and integrity. Topical corticosteroids can be selectively used if there are inflamed areas of skin (i.e., pink or red, not just dry and scaly). For many over-the-counter, all-purpose moisturizers, an inverse correlation between efficacy and cost has been demonstrated.

Prognosis

This condition tends to be chronic, but can be effectively treated with the above measures.

Key Points

- Xerotic dermatitis is a common and chronic condition in the elderly that is defined as dry, itchy skin.
- Consistent use of appropriate dry skin care regimens that include moisturizers and gentle cleansers is the cornerstone of management.

References

Judge MR, McLean WHI, Munro CS. Disorders of keratinization. In: Burns T, Breathnach S, Cox N, Griffiths C, editors. Rook's textbook of dermatology. 8th ed. Oxford: Wiley-Blackwell; 2010.

Norman RA. Xerosis and pruritus in the elderly: recognition and management. Dermatol Ther. 2003;16:254–9.

Proksch E, Lachapelle J-M. The management of dry skin with topical emollients – recent perspectives. J Dtsch Dermatolo Ges. 2005;3: 768–74.

Rapini RP, Bolognia JL, Jorizzo JL. Dermatology, vol. 2-volume set. St. Louis: Mosby; 2007.

Schafer-Korting M, Korting HC, Braun-Palco O. Liposome preparations: a step forward in topical drug therapy for skin disease? J Am Acad Derrnatol. 1989;21:1271.

Van Scott EJ, Yu RJ. Control of keratinization with alpha-hydroxy acids and related compounds. Arch Dermatol. 1974;110:586.

Wehr R, Krochmal L, Bagatell F, et al. A controlled two center study of ammonium lactate 12 percent lotion and a petrolatum-based creme in patients with xerosis. Cutis. 1986;37:205.

Chapter 23
70 Year Old Patient with Plaques

A 70 year-old white male presents to the office for the treatment of chronic psoriasis of 30 years. He has been really stressed recently due to his sister's hospitalization. In the past, he was treated with fluocinolone cream, calcipotriene (Dovonex), halcinonide (Halog), and UV light but they only relieved the symptoms temporarily. He had joint stiffness in the hips, knees, and fingers. It was worse in the morning and improved with activity.

On physical exam, the plaques were dry, silvery, and scaly and affected close to half his body surface area. Some of the plaques had excoriations and bleeding due to scratching (Fig. 23.1).

Based on the case description and the photograph, what is your diagnosis?

1. Eczema
2. Lichen simplex chronicus
3. Mycosis fungoides
4. Psoriasis

Diagnosis

Psoriasis

R.A. Norman, J. Endo, *Clinical Cases in Geriatric Dermatology*, Clinical Cases in Dermatology, DOI 10.1007/978-1-4471-4135-8_23, © Springer-Verlag London 2013

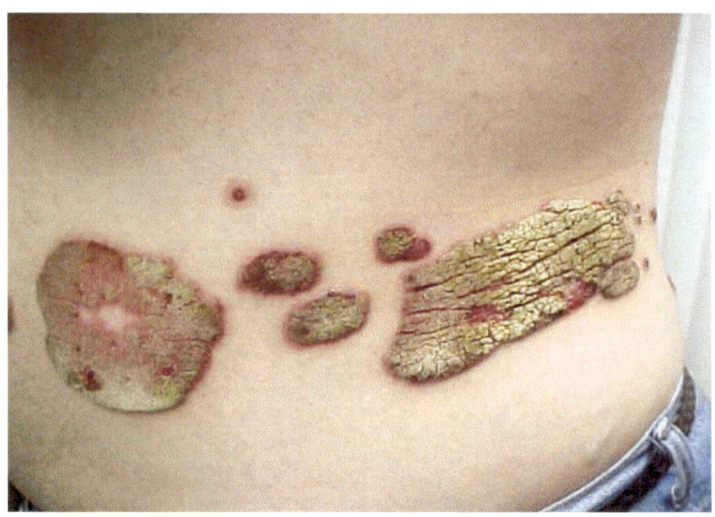

Figure 23.1 A 70 year-old male had extensive plaques with excoriations and bleeding due to scratching

Discussion

Psoriasis is a chronic, relapsing condition that affects 1–3 % of the population worldwide. The plaques are dry, red, and often described as having silvery-white scale that bleed when scratched. It most commonly affects the extensor surfaces of knees, elbows, scalp, toenails. It sometimes affects the face (sebopsoriasis), or palms and soles of the feet (palmoplantar pustulosis). Psoriasis is categorized as mild (<5 % of the body), moderate (5–30 % of the body), and severe (>30 % of the body). It is physically and emotionally debilitating in that a person's self confidence is affected due to the presence of plaques on the skin (Krueger 2005).

There are numerous factors that can exacerbate psoriasis. These include stress, trauma, systemic steroids (may cause flares after tapering). Smoking, obesity, and alcohol use are associated with psoriasis. Researchers at the University of Pennsylvania have found that even after adjusting for these traditional cardiovascular risk factors, psoriasis independently appears to be associated with excessive cardiovascular disease risk (Mehta 2011).

Therapies directed against cutaneous psoriasis are not curative, but rather keep the disease in remission. Treatments should be individualized to the type and severity of the disease as well as the patient's comorbidities. For patients who have mild psoriasis, the first line of treatment is topical agents, including topical steroids, calcipotriene (Dovonex), Anthralin, coal tar, PUVA, narrow band UVB, and intralesional steroids injections (Mason et al. 2009). For more severe or refractory disease, oral therapies include methotrexate and cyclosporine. Injectable biologic treatments, such as alefacept (Amevive), which interrupts T-cell interactions; and ustekinumab (Stelara), which has anti-Th17 activity, are other options.

Between 5–8 % of patients will develop psoriatic arthritis, and it affects men and women equally. It often manifests years after cutaneous psoriasis. Common symptoms include morning stiffness, or arthritis. When psoriatic arthritis is present, tumor necrosis factor (TNF) antagonists such as etanercept (Enbrel), adalimumab (Humira), and infliximab (Remicade) can be used. TNF antagonists should not be used in patients with severe congestive heart failure, history of autoimmune conditions (e.g., lupus, multiple sclerosis), or recent malignancy.

Other treatments for psoriatic arthritis include nonsteroidal anti-inflammatory drugs (NSAIDS), sulfasalazine, methotrexate, azathioprine, and leflunomide.

Our patient was prescribed etanercept (Enbrel) after a clear chest x-ray, normal liver enzymes, and negative hepatitis panel. At her 6 week follow-up, she reported 90 % improvement of psoriatic plaques of her legs, 60 % decreased in back lesions, and 40 % reductions of lesions throughout the body.

Key Points

- Psoriasis is an inflammatory skin condition that can also affect the nails and joints.

- Treatment depends upon the extent and severity of skin lesions as well as the presence of psoriatic arthritis (which can evolve after the cutaneous lesions).
- Psoriatic patients should be counseled about the recent data suggesting excessive risk of cardiovascular disease and need for screening and preventive measures.

References

Krueger JG, Bowcock A. Psoriasis pathophysiology: curent concepts of pathogenesis. Ann Rheum Dis. 2005;64 Suppl 2:ii30–6.

Mason AR, Mason J, Cork M, Dooley G, Edwards G. Topical treatments for chronic plaque psoriasis. Cochrane Database Syst Rev. 2009; Apr 15, CD005028.

Mehta NN, Yu Y, Pinnelas R, Krishnamoorthy P, Shin DB, Troxel AB, Gelfand JM. Attributable risk estimate of severe psoriasis on major cardiovascular events. Am J Med. 2011;124(8):775. e1–6.

Chapter 24
Man with Ruddy Cheeks and Big Red Nose

A 60 year-old white male presents with a several year history of a rash on his nose and cheeks that comes and goes. It worsens when he is outside mowing the lawn. He is embarrassed because several of his neighbors and friends have asked whether he was intoxicated. He has tried over-the-counter acne medications and washes, but nothing has improved his condition. He also complains that these medications have made his face dry and irritated.

On physical examination, the nose and bilateral cheeks are erythematous and dry with scattered telangiectasias as well as papules and pustules. His nose is slightly bulbous. There were no comedones present and his eyes were unaffected. (Fig. 24.1)

Based on the case description and the photograph, what is your diagnosis?

1. Acne vulgaris
2. Rosacea
3. Seborrheic dermatitis
4. Keratosis pilaris
5. Lupus erythematosus

R.A. Norman, J. Endo, *Clinical Cases in Geriatric Dermatology,* Clinical Cases in Dermatology, DOI 10.1007/978-1-4471-4135-8_24, © Springer-Verlag London 2013

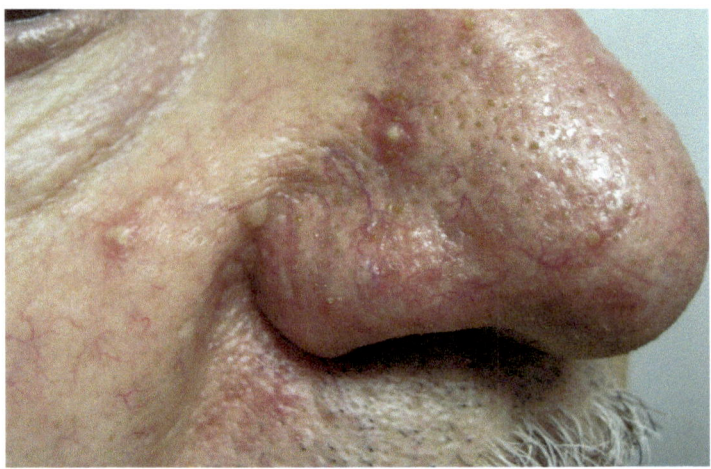

FIGURE 24.1 A 60 year-old white male presents with telangiectasias, papules, pustules and dryness on his cheeks and nose

Diagnosis

Rosacea

Discussion

Rosacea is a chronic disorder that most commonly affects the face. Several variants exist that often overlap. One is the erythematotelangiectatic type, characterized by redness and telangiectasias but no warmth to palpation. Another is papulopustular, which is frequently misdiagnosed as acne vulgaris (Crawford et al. 2004). Rhinophyma is a thickening of the skin of the nose that results in a larger and bulbous shape. Some patients develop ocular rosacea, which causes eye redness and irritation. Some rosacea patients develop psychological conditions like depression because of their negative self image (Craft et al. 2010).

Patients should avoid triggering factors, which include sun exposure, alcohol or spicy food ingestion, and overheating. Medical treatments include topical metronidazole or azelaic acid to reduce the swelling and redness. Tetracycline antibiotics are very effective in reducing the inflammation and redness as well as eye symptoms. Rhinophyma or large telangiectasias often require cosmetic procedures such as laser or pulsed-dye laser or surgery to correct.

Acne vulgaris – "teenage" acne is notable for the presence of comedones (blackheads and whiteheads). The inflammatory papules are usually more tender than in rosacea. Compared to the ones in rosacea. Patients suffering from acne do not develop rhinophyma.

Seborrheic dermatitis – The skin peels and yellow greasy scales are present particularly in otherwise oily areas of the body. Pustules are not present.

Keratosis pilaris – This is a condition in which the skin is dry and spiny plugs are formed in the hair follicles. The skin will look like "goosebumps" on the upper outer part of the arms and thighs. Telangiectasias are not characteristic.

Lupus erythematosus – The rash of acute systemic lupus is classically described as a butterfly rash on the malar cheeks and nose. It worsens with sun exposure, but does not have papules, pustules, telangiectasias.

Key Points

- Rosacea is a common inflammatory skin condition of adults, which can include flushing, telangiectasias, pustules, inflammatory papules. There is a notable absence of comedones. Rhinophyma sometimes occurs.
- Some rosacea patients develop ocular symptoms, which are generally treated with oral tetracycline family antibiotics or warm compresses and eye scrubs.

References

Craft N, et al. Rosacea. VisualDx Essential Adult Dermatol. 2010; 196–8. http://www.visualdx.com/essential-dermatology/adult.

Crawford GH, Pelle MT, James WD. Rosacea: I. Etiology, pathogenesis, and subtype classification. J Am Acad Dermatol. 2004;51(3):327–41. quiz 342–4.

Chapter 25
71 Year Old with Dry, Scaly Arms and Legs

A 71 year old Caucasian male presented to the office with a complaint of dry, scaly areas. Both his legs were covered in scattered and coalesced brown macules along with a dry scaly rash that continued from just below the knee all the way to his toes (Figs. 25.1, 25.2, and 25.3). He said that his skin color changes were not itchy, but made him feel self-conscious and he had decided not to wear shorts. The scaly rash on his legs did itch.

The patient stated that he had a heart attack several years ago and later noticed the beginnings of this brown color change.

Based on the case description and the photograph, what is your diagnosis?

1. Schamberg's disease
2. Stasis dermatitis
3. Lichen aureus
4. Gougerot-Blum disease
5. Majocchi's disease

Diagnosis

Schamberg's disease superimposed upon stasis dermatitis

R.A. Norman, J. Endo, *Clinical Cases in Geriatric Dermatology,* Clinical Cases in Dermatology, DOI 10.1007/978-1-4471-4135-8_25, © Springer-Verlag London 2013

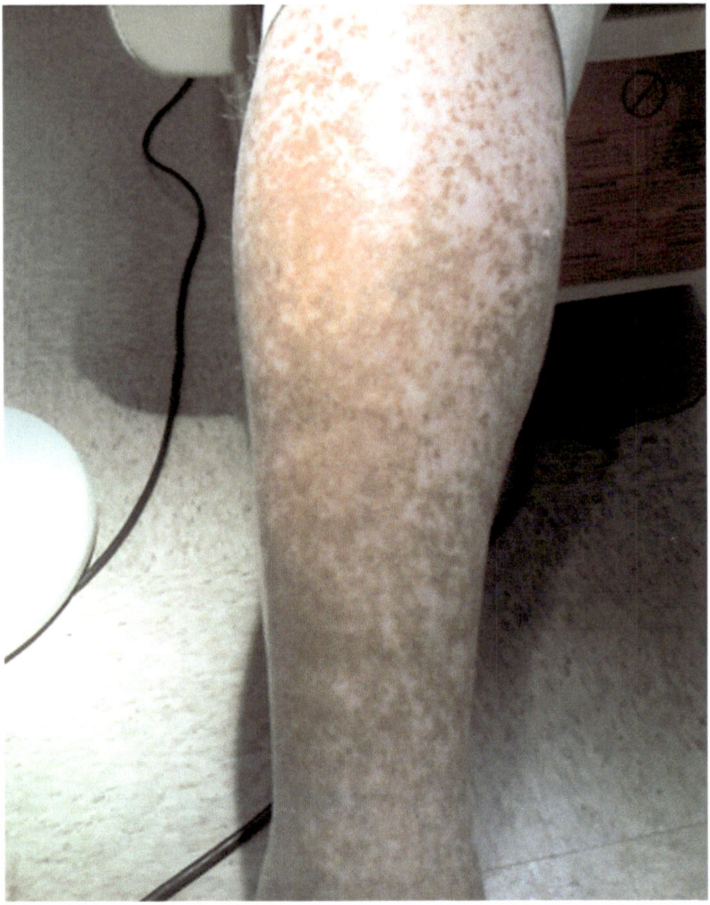

FIGURE 25.1 A 71 year old Caucasian male presented to the office with a complaint of dry, scaly brown macules

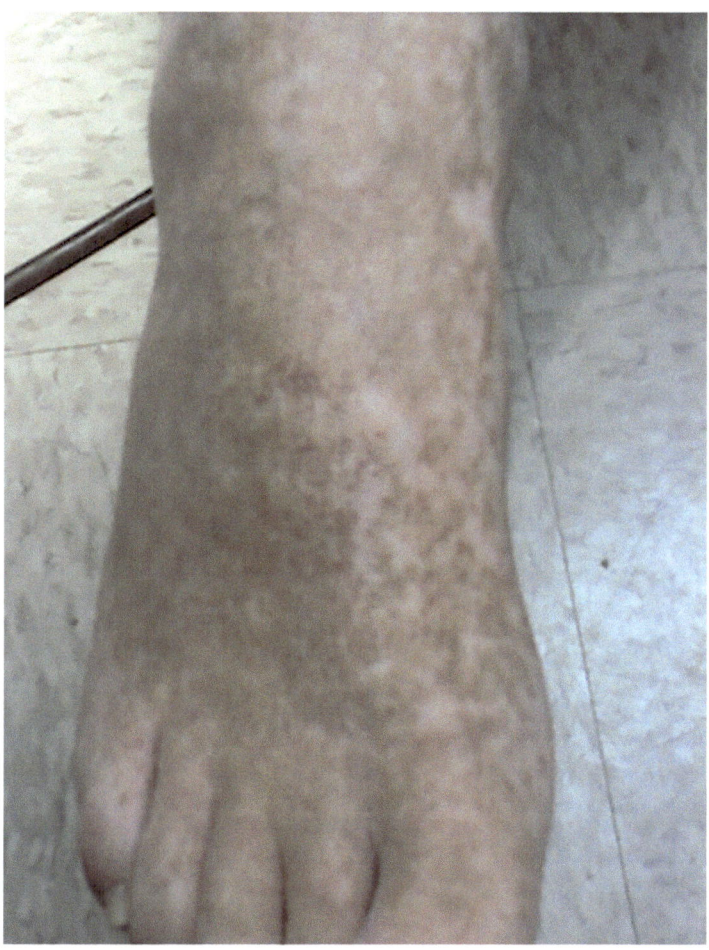

FIGURE 25.2 Both legs were covered in scattered and coalesced brown macules along with a dry scaly rash that continued from just below the knee all the way to his toes

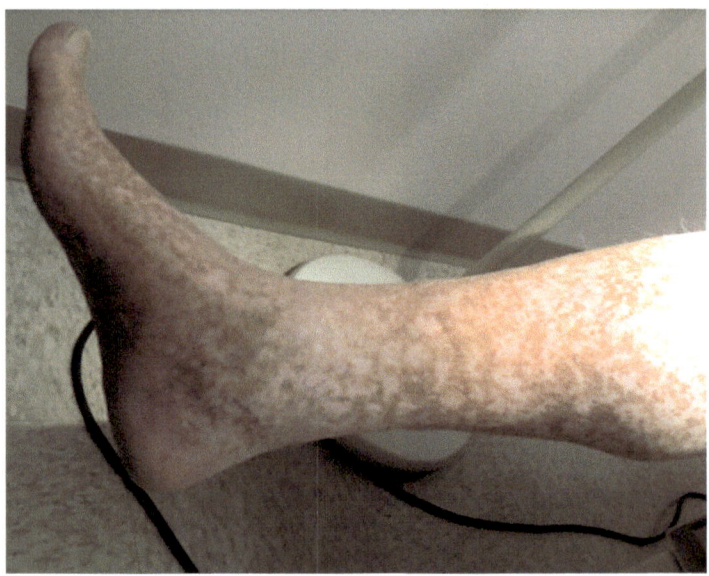

Figure 25.3 Both legs were covered in scattered and coalesced brown macules along with a dry scaly rash that continued from just below the knee all the way to his toes

Discussion

Schamberg's disease is a progressive purpuric dermatosis that is characterized by flat, petechial hemorrhages. This disease is seen in children and on the lower legs of older men. Schamberg's disease presents as lesions that are irregular patches red and brown in color with superimposed pinpoint cayenne pepper macules. The discoloration is due to the leakage of blood from small blood vessels near the skin surface. The red lesions are newer hemorrhages and the older lesions are brown from the hemosiderin deposits from the degradation of the extravascular erythrocytes. Sometimes the lesions can cause itching and discomfort (Ball et al. 2003; Bolognia et al. 2003).

There are several other types of pigmented purpuric dermatoses. Majocchi's disease is an annular variant that has telangiectasias. Gougerot-Blum disease has lesions of Schamberg's disease along with lichenoid papules, plaques, and macules. Lichen aureus has few patches that are rust colored, purple, or golden which arise from the extremities or from the trunk (Johnson et al. 2005).

Stasis dermatitis is a chronic venous insufficiency disease that causes peripheral edema, hyperpigmentation, fibrosis of the skin and subcutaneous tissue, and ulceration. Stasis dermatitis treatment options include elevation of the legs, the use of support hose, and topical corticosteroid medications. This patient's heart attack likely contributed to the addition of stasis dermatitis superimposed on his diagnosis of Schamberg's disease.

Key Points

- Progressive pigmented eruptions are benign rashes caused by capillaritis.
- Several clinical variants exist. Unless they are symptomatic, no specific therapy is warranted or consistently curative.

References

Ball JW, Benedict GW, Daines JE, Seidel HM. Mosby's guide to physical examination. 5th ed. St. Louis: Mosby; 2003. p. 163–224.

Bolognia JL, Jorizzo JL, Rapini RP. Dermatology, vol. 1. London: Mosby; 2003. p. 361–3.

Johnson RA, Suurmond D, Klaus W. Fitzpatrick's color atlas & synopsis of clinical dermatology. 5th ed. New York: McGraw-Hill; 2005. p. 136–7.

Chapter 26
76 Year Old Man with Chronic Rash

A 76-year-old man presents with a chief complaint of a chronic rash on the arms.

On examination you observe multiple irregular, eroded, infiltrated papules on the arms in various stages. (Fig. 26.1) There are several old scars and significant lichenification (skin thickening). Similar lesions are not present at other skin sites.

Based on the case description and the photograph, what is your diagnosis?

1. Basal cell carcinoma
2. Squamous cell carcinoma
3. Contact dermatitis
4. Prurigo nodularis

Diagnosis

Prurigo nodularis

R.A. Norman, J. Endo, *Clinical Cases in Geriatric Dermatology,* Clinical Cases in Dermatology, DOI 10.1007/978-1-4471-4135-8_26, © Springer-Verlag London 2013

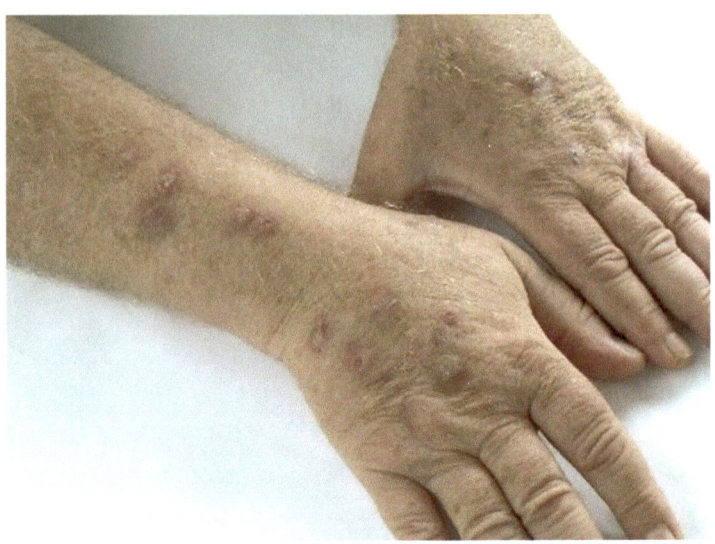

FIGURE 26.1 A 76-year-old man presented with a chronic rash on the arms

Discussion

Prurigo nodularis is a localized form of neurodermatitis, which may be secondary to habitual and often almost unconscious scratching (Doyle et al. 1979).

This dermatitis was treated with a topical corticosteroid ointment preparation with a covering to minimize scratching and improve penetration of the medication.

Consider prurigo nodularis in situations with a localized cluster of infiltrated, crusted papules in areas that are easily scratched (Lee 2005). The face, palms, and soles are rarely affected and the sparing of the mid upper back due to the inability to reach this area is referred to as the "butterfly sign." It is presumably caused by constant picking or scratching.

Symptomatic treatment includes anti-pruritics and moisturizers, oral anti-histamines, and phototherapy. Doxepin or mirtazapine can be helpful (Fried 2003; Grillo et al. 2007).

Scabies also causes extreme pruritus and crusted papules. However, it would be unusual to have severe localized disease and not lesions elsewhere. A skin scraping can be performed to look for scabies.

Insect bite reaction can produce multiple clustered papules on the arms, although this would be a fairly uncommon location and the chronic nature of the process makes this very unlikely.

Basal cell carcinoma and squamous cell carcinoma may cause eroded or ulcerated, irregular papules. It would be unusual to have this many lesions in the same general area without some underlying factor, such as previous radiation, to the site.

Contact dermatitis to material applied to the site can result in lichenification and crusting. However, it would not cause discrete substantive papules, as in this case.

Key Points

- Prurigo nodularis is caused by chronic rubbing, picking, or scratching of the skin.
- If no underlying cause of pruritus is found, symptomatic treatment options can be tried.

References

Doyle JA, Connolly SM, Hunziker N, Winkelmann RK. Prurigo nodularis: a reappraisal of the clinical and histologic features. J Cutan Pathol. 1979;6:392–403.

Fried R, Fried S. Picking apart the picker: a clinician's guide for management of the patient presenting with excoriations. Psychocutan Med. 2003;71:291–8.

Grillo M, Long R, Long D. Habit reversal training for the itch scratch cycle associated with pruritic skin conditions. Dermatol Nurs. 2007;19(3):243–8.

Lee MR, Shumack S. Prurigo nodularis: a review. Australas J Dermatol. 2005;46(4):211–8.

Chapter 27
Enlarging Plaques on the Left Leg

64-year-old woman presents with a 3-year history of two gradually enlarging, asymptomatic lesions of the left leg.

On examination you observe two distinct, annular (advancing margin and central clearing) plaques with a thready border and minimal erythema at the bases. There are no papules or vesicles on the borders (Fig. 27.1).

Based on the case description and the photograph, what is your diagnosis?

1. Tinea corporis
2. Granuloma annulare
3. Annular sarcoidosis
4. Erythema annulare centrifugum
5. Porokeratosis

Diagnosis

Porokeratosis

R.A. Norman, J. Endo, *Clinical Cases in Geriatric Dermatology,* Clinical Cases in Dermatology, DOI 10.1007/978-1-4471-4135-8_27, © Springer-Verlag London 2013

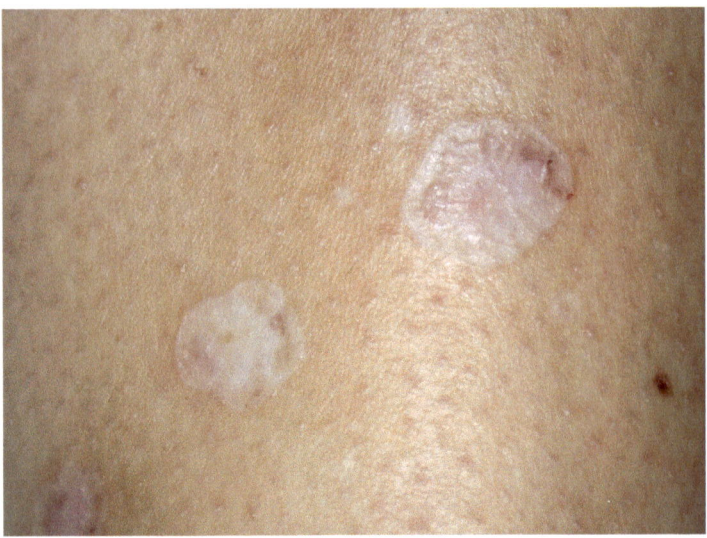

FIGURE 27.1 A 64-year-old woman with thready bordered thin plaques

Discussion

Porokeratosis is a benign clonal disorder of keratinization that results in a thready scale on the advancing border of one or more skin lesions (Freedberg 2003; James et al. 2005; Judge et al. 2010). In geriatric patients, the most common variant is disseminated superficial actinic porokeratosis (DSAP). Treatment options are numerous and often unsuccessful. Our patient had cryosurgery but was lost to follow up.

Tinea corporis is typically annular and has a scaly border. The thin, thready border is somewhat atypical, but a microscopic examination or culture would be needed to absolutely rule this out.

Granuloma annulare produces one or more annular plaques which often appear on the hands. With rare exceptions, a thready, scaly border is not seen in this purely dermal disease.

Annular sarcoidosis occasionally has scale on the border of the lesions, but seldom appears as a solitary plaque on the leg.

Erythema annulare centrifugum is one of the figurate erythemas which represents a hypersensitivity reaction to malignancy, infection, or drugs. It has an annular configuration and is scaly at the border, but the scale trails after the advancing red rim rather than being on it.

Key Points

- Consider porokeratosis if there are annular plaques with a thin, thready, scaly border on sun-exposed skin.
- Treatment options are numerous, though many are unsuccessful.

References

Freedberg IM, et al. Fitzpatrick's dermatology in general medicine. 6th ed. New York: McGraw-Hill; 2003.

James W, Berger T, Elston D. Andrews' diseases of the skin: clinical dermatology. 10th ed. Philadelphia: Saunders; 2005.

Judge MR, McLean WHI, Munro CS. Disorders of keratinization. In: Burns T, Breathnach S, Cox N, Griffiths C, editors. Rook's textbook of dermatology. 8th ed. Oxford: Wiley-Blackwell; 2010.

Chapter 28
76 Year Old with a Shallow Ulcer

A 76-year-old patient with history of hypertension and varicose veins presented with indurated and hyperpigmented skin of the lower legs and a shallow ulcer on the left medial malleolus (Fig. 28.1).

Based on the case description and the photograph, what is your diagnosis?

1. Venous stasis (gravitational) ulcer
2. Hypertensive (arterial) ulcer
3. Atrophie blanche
4. Neoplastic ulcer
5. Infectious ulcer

Diagnosis

Venous stasis (gravitational) ulcer

Discussion

Chronic venous disease is the most common cause of lower leg ulcers (Bolognia 2008). Venous stasis ulcers typically occur on the medial malleoli (ankles) and legs, with concomitant stasis dermatitis, macules, papules, varicose veins, cyanosis, dependent

R.A. Norman, J. Endo, *Clinical Cases in Geriatric Dermatology,* Clinical Cases in Dermatology, DOI 10.1007/978-1-4471-4135-8_28, © Springer-Verlag London 2013

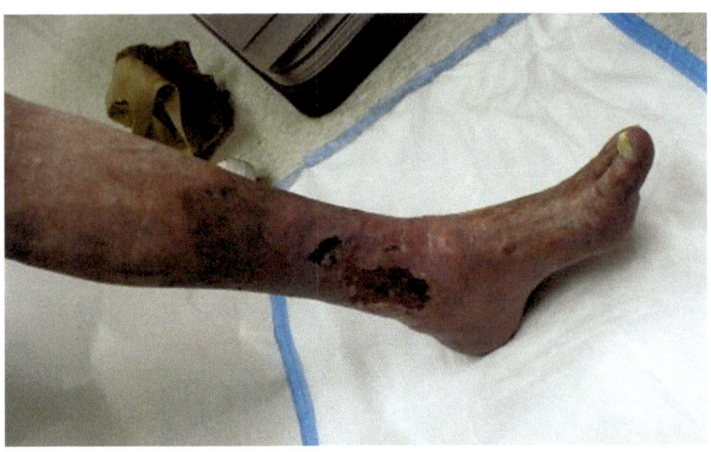

Figure 28.1 Indurated and hyperpigmented plaques of the lower legs and a shallow ulcer on the left medial malleolus

edema, and pain. There is often red-brown skin discoloration from hemosiderin deposition and induration. In severe end-stage cases, a panniculitis (lipodermatosclerosis) can develop with painful, indurated, scarred plaques.

Venous ulcers (venous hypertension ulcers or venous insufficiency ulcers) are caused by poor venous blood return from the legs to the heart. Several etiologies include inadequate calf muscle pump, incompetent venous valves, venous obstruction. Early venous stasis dermatitis of the legs results from tissue hypoxemia, extravasation of red blood cells, and iron (hemosiderin) deposition in the dermis. The affected area is at increased risk of developing contact dermatitis to topical medications such as neomycin, aloe vera, vitamin E, and benzocaine.

Hypertensive (arterial) ulcers usually present as clean, "punched-out" ulcers on the lateral malleoli and legs. There is often concomitant shiny skin, hair loss, pallor, and decreased pulses. Pain is relieved by dependency but exacerbated by leg elevation, in contrast to venous stasis ulcers (Preachey et al.

1986).

Atrophie blanche describes the porcelain white reticular scarring and atrophy, usually on the lower third of the calf, ankle, and dorsal foot. It is often associated with thrombotic vasculopathy, although other causes of leg ulceration can also lead to this finding (Shomick et al. 1983).

Neoplastic ulcer often occur at the site of a previous draining ulcer or burn scar. In addition to the prototypical example of Marjolin's ulcer with squamous cell, other tumors presenting with chronic ulceration can include mycosis fungoides, basal cell carcinoma (rodent ulcer), and keratoacanthoma. Nonhealing ulcers despite aggressive wound care should prompt the clinician to consider a biopsy to rule out underling malignancy.

Infectious ulcers can be caused by bacterial, fungal (chromoblastomycosis), treponemal, parasitic, and rarely viral (herpetic) pathogens.

Inflammatory ulcers can be produced by vasculitis of any cause, especially rheumatoid arthritis, diabetes (ulcerative necrobiosis lipoidica diabeticorum), panniculitis, and pyoderma gangrenosum.

Mal perforans occurs in diabetics whose lack of sensation predisposes to traumatic and vascular ulceration of the sole.

Traumatic or factitial ulcers often display bizarre, irregular shapes, and can occur wherever the patient can reach. These can occur from injecting drugs under the skin ("skin popping") or from underlying anxiety and depression, resulting in deep excoriations.

The underlying cause must be treated or eliminated (Falanga 1986). For venous stasis ulcers-soaks, leg elevation, compression stockings, Unna's boot (zinc oxide, glycerin, and gauze bandage). Referral to a vascular surgeon and vascular imaging should be considered in severe or recurrent cases. Medical therapy can include topical steroids and pentoxifylline (Trental), 400 mg orally BID (Velanovich 1990).

Key Points

- Chronic leg ulcers can be caused by many conditions, although venous ulcers account for the majority.
- Aggressive compressive therapy is the first-line treatment in prevent and treating venous stasis.
- For a chronic, nonhealing ulcer, biopsy should be considered to rule out occult malignancy.

References

Bolognia J, Jorizzo JL, Rapini RP. Dermatology. St. Louis: Mosby/Elsevier; 2008.

Falanga V, Baglstein WH. A therapeutic approach to venous ulcers. J Am Acad Dermatol. 1986;14:777.

Preachey RDG, Crissey JT. Leg ulcers. In: Rook A, Parish C, Beare JM, editors. Practical management of the dermatologic patient. Philadelphia: J. B. Lippincott; 1986. p. 213–5.

Shomick JK, Nicholas BK, Bergstresser PR, Gilliam JN. Idiopathic atrophie blanche. J Am Acad Dermatol. 1983;8:792.

Velanovich V, Fahey M. Treatment of ischemic leg ulcers with pentoxifylline: a case report and theoretical considerations. Ann Plast Surg. 1990;25:58–62.

Part V
Drug Eruptions

Chapter 29
Full Body Rash

A 57 year-old Caucasian patient presented to the office asking for evaluation of a full body rash that started approximately 9 weeks ago (Figs. 29.1, 29.2, and 29.3). The patient had a previously diagnosed acinic cancer, a rare salivary gland tumor, arising from his right neck. He had three surgeries for tumor recurrences. His chemotherapy included cisplatin, docetaxel, and most recently, cetuximab for the last 11 weeks. After the first 2 weeks of cetuximab, the patient noticed a pruritic, monomorphous popular and pustular rash spreading over his face, trunk, back, and arms. The lower extremities and the genitals have been spared.

Based on the case description and the photograph, what is your diagnosis?

1. Acneiform rash
2. Erythema multiforme
3. Hypersensitivity vasculitis
4. Stevens-Johnson syndrome

Diagnosis

Acneiform rash

R.A. Norman, J. Endo, *Clinical Cases in Geriatric Dermatology,* Clinical Cases in Dermatology, DOI 10.1007/978-1-4471-4135-8_29, © Springer-Verlag London 2013

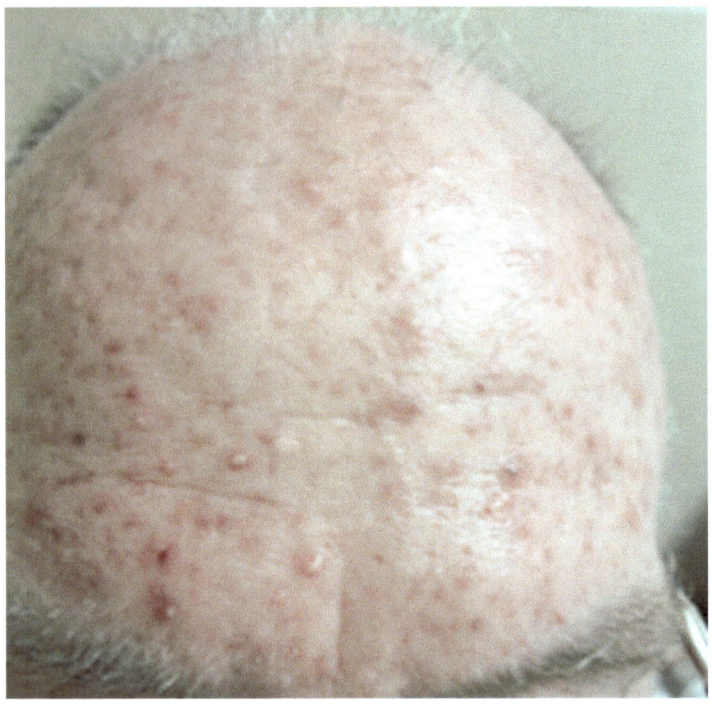

Figure 29.1 A 57 year-old Caucasian patient presented with full body rash that started after chemotherapy for a salivary gland tumor

Discussion

Cetuximab (Erbitux), is an intravenously administered monoclonal antibody that antagonizes epidermal growth factor receptors (EGFR) and is effective against metastatic diseases (Balagula et al. 2011). It is effective against metastatic colorectal and head/neck cancers because EGFR is typically overexpressed in these tumors (Bonner 2010). Most EGFR inhibitors cause adverse cutaneous reactions with the most frequently reported being acneiform eruption: follicular based macules, papules, or pustules (Tomková et al. 2010). It should be noted that the rash is not a drug hypersensitivity; therefore, it is not an

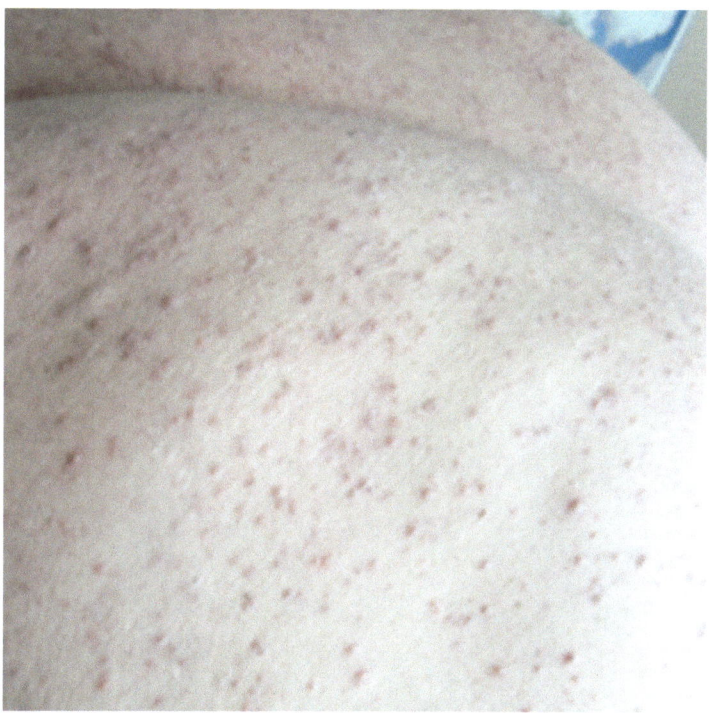

FIGURE 29.2 A 57 year-old Caucasian patient with a generalized follicular-based eruption after initiation chemotherapy for a recurrent salivary gland tumor

indication to discontinue treatment (Lynch et al. 2007). Other skin related side effects of cetuximab include eczema, hyperpigmentation, conjunctivitis, telangiectasias, fissures, desquamation, paranoychia, xerosis, and destruction of both hair and nails (DeWitt et al. 2007).

EGFR is expressed in the epidermis and hair follicles Receptor antagonism therefore disrupts proliferation and differentiation causing abnormal alterations in skin structures and the release of inflammatory mediators (Lenz 2006).

There is some controversy about acneiform reactions predicting antitumor effect. For example, Tomková et al. found

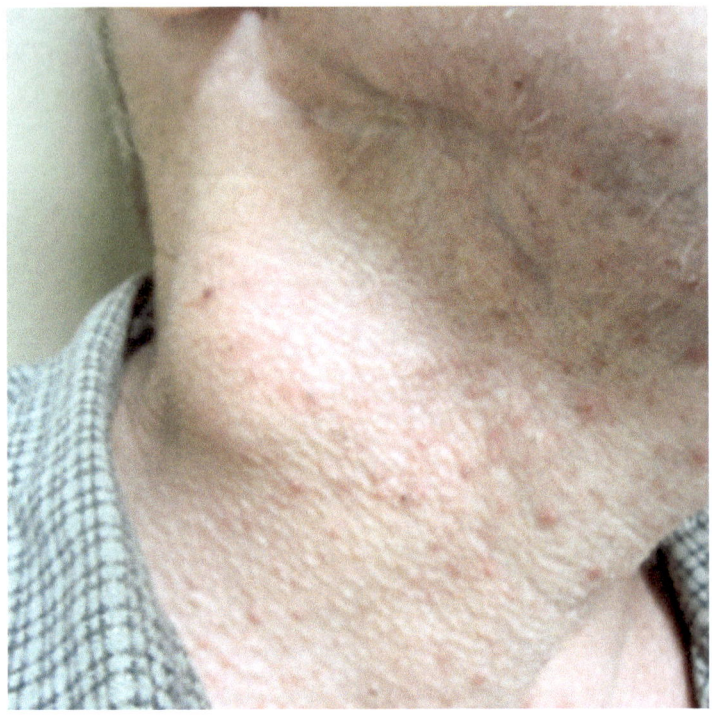

FIGURE 29.3 Patient presenting with follicular-based eruption after starting chemotherapy for a rare salivary gland tumor (notice neck mass)

no relationship between the severity of the acneiform rash and the patient's cancer outcome. However, Bonner et al. reported that patients with severe cetuximab-induced rashes, there was a better 5-year survival rate than patients with mild or no rashes at all.

Biopsy of the acneiform rash typically displays characteristic perifollicular lymphoneutrophilic infiltrate within the epidermis and adnexal structures.

Drug cessation or even dosage reduction is typically not needed. Several studies have demonstrated the success traditional acne treatments in treating the eruption, such as topical adapalene, oral isotretinoin, oral tetracyclines, emollients, and topical antibiotics. Some institutions use minocycline prophylactically and during cetuximab therapy (Boggs 2007; Dancey 2003). It is unknown whether treating the acneiform eruption modulates the chemotherapeutic tumor response.

Key Points

- Acneiform eruption can occur with epidermal growth factor receptor (EGFR) inhibitors, which are chemotherapeutic agents used in metastatic gastrointestinal and otolaryngological tumors.
- The presence of acneiform eruption during EGFR treatment might predict tumor response, although this is controversial.
- It is unknown whether treating the acneiform interferes with EGFR chemotherapeutic effect. Nonetheless, some institutions advocate for prophylactic acne treatment during EGFR treatment.

References

Balagula Y, Garbe C, Myskowski PL, Hauschild A, Rapoport BL, Boers-Doets CB, Lacouture ME. Clinical presentation and management of dermatological toxicities of epidermal growth factor receptor inhibitors. Int J Dermatol. 2011;50:129–46.

Boggs W. Oral minocycline reduces cetuximab-associated papular rash. J Clin Oncol. 2007;25:5390–6.

Bonner JA, Harari PM, Giralt J, Cohen RB, Jones CU, Sur RK, Raben D, Ang KK. Radiotherapy plus cetuximab for locoregionally advanced head and neck cancer: 5-year survival data from a phase 3 randomised trial, and relation between cetuximab-induced rash and survival. Lancet Oncol. 2010;11(1):21–8.

Dancey J, Sausville EA. Issues and progress with protein kinase inhibitors for cancer treatment. Nat Rev Drug Discov. 2003;2: 296–313.

DeWitt CA, Siroy AE, Stone SP. Acneiform eruptions associated with epidermal growth factor receptor-targeted chemotherapy. J Am Acad Dermatol. 2007;56(3):500–5.

Lenz HJ. Anti-EGFR mechanism of action: antitumor effect and underlying cause of adverse events. Oncology. 2006;20(5 Suppl 2): 5–13.

Lynch TJ, Kim ES, Eaby B, et al. Epidermal growth factor receptor inhibitor-associated cutaneous toxicities: an evolving paradigm in clinical management. Oncologist. 2007;12:610–21.

Tomková H, Kohoutek M, Zábojníková M, Pospíšková M, Ostřížková L, Gharibyar M. Cetuximab-induced cutaneous toxicity. J Eur Acad Dermatol Venereol. 2010;24:692–6.

Chapter 30
Itchy Edematous Papules

A 59 year old man comes in with 2 month history of itchy edematous papules (Figs. 30.1 and 30.2) that come and go in less than 24 hours.

Based on the case description and the photograph, what is your diagnosis?

1. Urticarial vasculitis
2. Bullous pemphigoid
3. Erythema multiforme
4. Angioedema
5. Urticaria

Diagnosis

Urticaria

Discussion

Urticaria is often described as pink, edematous dermal plaques and papules which often exhibit peripheral blanching and dermographism (wheal, flare, erythema-triple response of Lewis). Individual lesions characteristically wax, wane, and

R.A. Norman, J. Endo, *Clinical Cases in Geriatric Dermatology,* Clinical Cases in Dermatology, DOI 10.1007/978-1-4471-4135-8_30, © Springer-Verlag London 2013

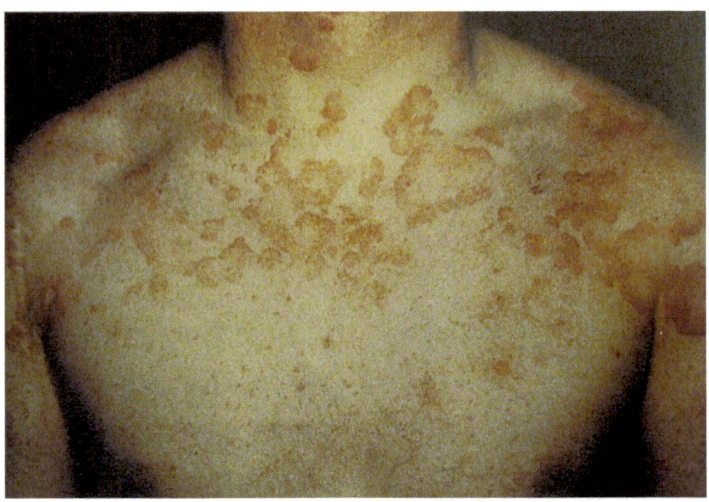

FIGURE 30.1 A 59 year old man comes in with 2 month history of itchy edematous papules on his chest

migrate in less than 24 h, often in less than an hour (Axelrod 2011; Deacock 2008; Grattan 2008; Kaplan 2009).

Allergic (IgE-mediated) or nonallergic (direct) mast cell degranulation results in histamine release, vasodilation, and dermal edema. Common causes include the following:

1. Drugs-penicillin, aspirin, morphine, iodine
2. Infections-Streptococcus, hepatitis B, parasitic infestations
3. Foods-seafood, citrus, berries, chocolate
4. Stings-Hymenoptera (bee, wasp)
5. Physical factors-increased body core temperature (cholinergic urticaria), cold physical pressure from tight clothing.
6. Contactants-chemicals can cause contact urticaria.

   Biopsy is usually not necessary or helpful except to rule out urticarial vasculitis (see below). The minimal changes of dermal edema may not be apparent during processing, especially if epinephrine-containing anesthetic is used during biopsy (Breathnach 2010).

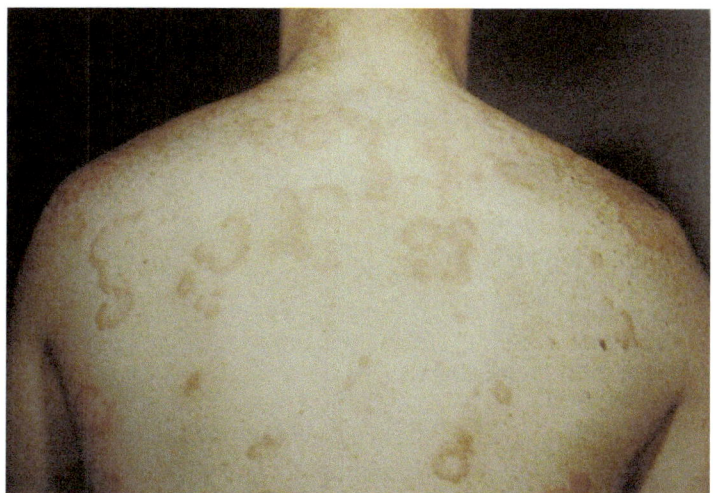

FIGURE 30.2 A 59 year old man comes in with 2 month history of itchy edematous annular papules on his back

Differentials:

1. Urticarial vasculitis-lesions persist for over 24 h as "fixed urticaria," may become hemorrhagic. Biopsy reveals a leukocytoclastic vasculitis.
2. Bullous pemphigoid-urticarial phase. In this variant, classic tense bullae are often absent. Clinical suspicion, non-response to antihistamines, and skin biopsy provide clues. Direct immunofluorescent or serologic studies can confirm the diagnosis.
3. Erythema multiforme. Targetoid lesions should be present with central epidermal change.
4. Angioedema-deep, subcutaneous urticaria that may affect the lips and throat; can be fatal (Kontou-Fili et al. 1997)

Treatment:

1. Search for and treat possible underlying causes.
2. High-dose antihistamines are more effective at preventing than relieving hives.

3. Subcutaneously administered epinephrine (Adrenalin) and other vasoconstrictors (Epi-Pen, ANA-Kit preloaded syringes) are prescribed to prevent anaphylactic shock. They are effective emergency treatments for hives and orolaryngeal angioedema.
4. Systemic corticosteroids suppress urticaria but must be used cautiously until infectious causes have been eliminated. They provide temporary relief only and should generally be avoided due to long-term side effects.
5. Heavy exercising, overheating, sweating, and the use of caffeine, alcohol, coffee, tea, and other hot beverages should be avoided. Also, wearing loose clothing is helpful to reduce the occurrence of pressure urticaria.
6. When urticaria becomes chronic (more than 6 weeks) and do not respond to antihistamines, a thorough history, examination, and laboratory evaluation should be considered. The reason being that if no reversible underlying cause can be found, systemic immunosuppressants are often the next tier of therapy (Powell et al. 2007).

Prognosis

Urticaria is often self-limited. In over 50 % of patients, no cause is detectable. Chronic urticaria (longer than 6 weeks) is especially difficult to treat, and often requires hospitalization, elimination diets, long-term antihistamines and immunosuppression, and environmental safeguards.

Key Points

• Urticaria are defined as hives lasting less than 24 hours. Lesions lasting longer, resolving with a bruise or associated with systemic symptoms warrant further evaluation to exclude urticarial vasculitis.
• A careful history can be helpful to find possible causes.

References

Axelrod S, Davis-Lorton M. Urticaria and angioedema. Mt Sinai J of Med: J Transl Personalized Med. 2011;78:784–802.

Breathnach SM. Drug reactions. In: Burns T, Breathnach S, Cox N, Griffiths C, editors. Rook's textbook of dermatology. 8th ed. Oxford: Wiley-Blackwell; 2010.

Deacock SJ. An approach to the patient with urticaria. Clin Exp Immunol. 2008;153:151–61.

Grattan CEH, Kobza Black A. Urticaria and mastocytosis. In: Burns T, Breathnach S, Cox N, Griffiths C, editors. Rook's textbook of dermatology. 7th ed. Malden: Blackwell Publishing, Inc.; 2008.

Kaplan AP. Urticaria and angioedema. In: Kay AB, Kaplan AP, Bousquet J, Holt PG, editors. Allergy and allergic diseases, vol. 2. 2nd ed. Oxford: Wiley-Blackwell; 2009.

Kontou-Fili K, Borici-Mazi R, Kapp A, Matjevic LJ, Mitchel FB. Physical urticaria: classification and diagnostic guidelines. Allergy. 1997;52:504–13.

Powell RJ, Du Toit GL, Siddique N, Leech SC, Dixon TA, Clark AT, Mirakian R, Walker SM, Huber PAJ, Nasser SM. BSACI guidelines for the management of chronic urticaria and angio-oedema. Clin Exp Allergy. 2007;37:631–50.

Part VI
Hair and Nails

Chapter 31
A 65 Year Old Female with Thinning Hair

A 65-year-old female presenting with a several-decade history of asymptomatic thinning hair on the scalp. The patient had no antecedent illnesses or change in medications or new hair styling products. No treatments have been prescribed yet to date. The remainder of her past history is negative. Of note, she thinks that her maternal grandmother might have also had some thinning starting in middle age.

Examination

There is decreased hair density on the parietal scalp and also near the crown with retention of the frontal hairline and the occipital hairs. Several short, thin-caliber hairs are found within the areas of alopecia (Fig. 31.1). Eyebrows, eyelashes and the remainder of body hair are intact. There is no inflammation, scale or scarring. Firm hair pull test yields two telogen hair shafts.

Based on the case description and the photograph, what is your diagnosis:

1. Alopecia areata.
2. Syphilis.
3. Androgenetic alopecia.

R.A. Norman, J. Endo, *Clinical Cases in Geriatric Dermatology,* Clinical Cases in Dermatology,
DOI 10.1007/978-1-4471-4135-8_31,
© Springer-Verlag London 2013

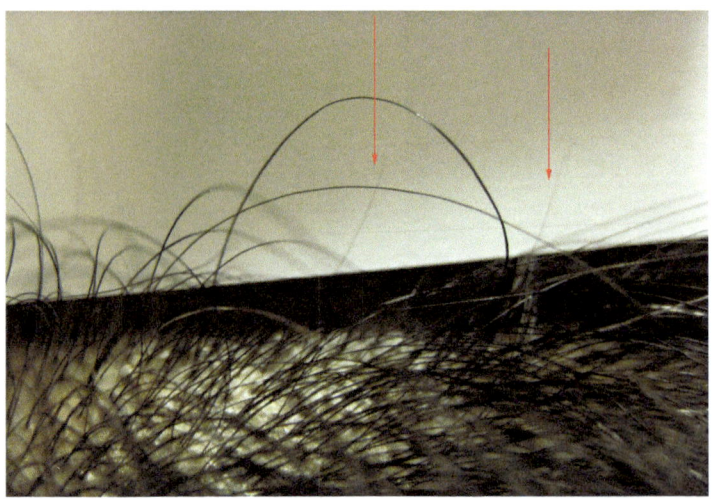

FIGURE 31.1 Female patient complaining of alopecia with several short, thin-caliber hairs (*red arrows*) near the vertex and mid scalp

4. Telogen effluvium.
5. Trichotillomania.

Diagnosis

Androgenetic alopecia.

Discussion

Androgenetic alopecia (AGA) is a common entity in both men and women. Classically, it begins as early as the late teens or early 20s all the way until middle-age. Contrary to popular belief, AGA is not exclusively found in men or those with a family history of balding in male relatives. In men, the classic pattern of hair loss is recession of the temples and vertex. In women, the frontal hairline is usually preserved with diffuse involvement spanning from the parietal scalp to the crown (Blume-Peytavi et al. 2011). There is ongoing controversy whether AGA is a risk marker of underlying conditions such as impaired fasting glucose and prostate cancer (Acibucu et al. 2010; Cremers et al. 2010; Abdel Fattah & Darwish 2011; Yassa et al. 2011).

The pathophysiology in men is hypothesized to be caused by a genetic predisposition of affected hair follicles to have increased activity of type II 5-alpha reductase (Blume-Peytavi et al. 2011). In women, the exact cause is less clear. Clinically and histologically, miniaturized hairs are seen, which are shorter in length and narrower in caliber compared to normal hairs. Histologically, androgenic alopecia and normal senescent alopecia in patients 60 and older are indistinguishable. However, recent microarray data by Mirmirani et al. suggest these are two distinct entities that should be treated differently (Mirmirani et al. 2007).

Hair loss is insidious and is not necessarily constant in rate. It may or may not be associated with mild pruritus or scalp dysesthesia, though there is a notable absence of inflammation and scarring. Areas outside the scalp are not involved (Blume-Peytavi et al. 2011). The hair pull test is considered positive when fewer than four telogen hairs (clubbed roots) are removed with a gentle tug and is highly suggestive of telogen effluvium (Blumeyer et al. 2011).

Because this condition is chronic and seems to be genetically programmed, the patients need to be on indefinite medical treatment to maintain hair. The first line of treatment is topical minoxidil. At this time, 5 % strength is FDA-approved for men only and 2 % for women. Although the solution vehicle is generic and cheaper than the branded Rogaine foam, the former contains propylene glycol and tends to cause irritant dermatitis (Bolognia et al. 2008). The medication should be applied directly to the scalp when dry rather than the hairs and must be used on a twice daily basis indefinitely. Second line treatment includes oral finasteride 1 mg daily (Propecia), which is an 5-alpha reductase inhibitor. This is only FDA-approved for men (Bolognia et al. 2008). Patient should be counseled that medical therapy takes several months to notice improvement and that upon stopping therapy, any hairs they would have otherwise lost because of their genetic predisposition will thin.

Hair transplant may be offered to patients, although it is generally recommended that the patient be on medical therapy before entertaining this procedure (Bolognia et al. 2008). It requires skilled technicians and significant time and expertise to achieve an excellent cosmetic outcome.

Differential Diagnoses

1. Syphilis has a classically moth-eaten appearance that is more patchy (Blumeyer et al. 2011). Sexual history, other review of systems, and serologic tests are useful in detecting this condition.
2. Alopecia areata is an autoimmune-driven form of alopecia that presents with abrupt onset of well-demarcated patches of non-scarring alopecia without miniaturization. Pigmented hairs seem to be more affected earlier in the disease process, leading to "overnight" greying. Close inspection of hairs adjacent to the border of the alopecia patch sometimes demonstrates "exclamation point" hairs that have a narrower caliber proximally and normal caliber distally. The disease can involve any hair-bearing skin. Nail pitting is sometimes also found (Bolognia et al. 2008). This entity is often self-remitting and can be associated with other autoimmune conditions such as thyroid disease, diabetes and vitiligo (Blumeyer et al. 2011).
3. Telogen effluvium is a non-scarring alopecia that classically follows 3 months after a major illness, stress, or surgery. There is disruption of the hair growth cycle without scalp inflammation, and hair loss tends to be diffuse. Hair regrowth occurs several months after recovery from the initial inciting event (Blumeyer et al. 2011).
4. Trichotillomania is habitual picking and twisting of hairs as either a habit or associated with an underlying psychiatric condition. Hair loss tends to be irregular, and broken off hairs of various lengths can be noted (Bolognia et al. 2008). Treatment with behavioral modification, coping skill teaching, or selective serotonin reuptake inhibitors (SSRIs) are sometimes helpful (Blumeyer et al. 2011).

Key Points

- Androgenetic alopecia (AGA) is characterized by miniaturized hairs with or without family history of hair loss.
- First-line treatment is topical minoxidil, with the foam vehicle being less likely to cause irritant scalp dermatitis.
- Areas of controversy include the possible association of AGA with other metabolic diseases and whether it is pathophysiologically distinct from senescent alopecia.

References

Abdel Fattah NS, Darwish YW. Androgenetic alopecia and insulin resistance: are they truly associated? Int J Dermatol. 2011;50:417–22.

Acibucu F, Kayatas M, Candan F. The association of insulin resistance and metabolic syndrome in early androgenetic alopecia. Singapore Med J. 2010;51:931–6.

Blume-Peytavi U, Blumeyer A, Tosti A, Finner A, Marmol V, Trakatelli M, et al. S1 guideline for diagnostic evaluation in androgenetic alopecia in men, women and adolescents. Br J Dermatol. 2011;164:5–15.

Blumeyer A, Tosti A, Messenger A, Reygagne P, Del Marmol V, Spuls PI, et al. Evidence-based (S3) guideline for the treatment of androgenetic alopecia in women and in men. J Dtsch Dermatol Ges. 2011;9 Suppl 6:S1-57. Journal of the German Society of Dermatology.

Bolognia J, Jorizzo JL, Rapini RP. Dermatology. St. Louis: Mosby/Elsevier; 2008.

Cremers RG, Aben KK, Vermeulen SH, den Heijer M, van Oort IM, Kiemeney LA. Androgenic alopecia is not useful as an indicator of men at high risk of prostate cancer. Eur J Cancer. 2010;46:3294–9. Oxford, England: 1990.

Mirmirani P, Oshtory S, Daoud S, McCormick T, Cooper K, Karnik P. Distinct patterns of gene expression in androgenetic and senescent alopecia – a microarray-based study. Fifth International Congress of Hair Research Societies. Vancouver, Canada, 2007.

Yassa M, Saliou M, De Rycke Y, Hemery C, Henni M, Bachaud JM, et al. Male pattern baldness and the risk of prostate cancer. Ann Oncol. 2011;22:1824–7. official journal of the European Society for Medical Oncology/ESMO.

Chapter 32
A 68-Year-Old Man with Brittle Nails

This elderly gentleman presents with progressively brittle nails that tend to break very easily (Fig. 32.1). He has no past history of other medical problems, and denies any history of nutritional deficiencies.

Upon examination, you notice all of his fingernails and toenails are thin and a few have splitting within the distal nail plate.

Based on the case description and the photograph what is your diagnosis?

1. Psoriatic nail disease
2. Onychomycosis
3. Senescent nail disease with possible superimposed irritant nail disease
4. Pterygium from lichen planus
5. Median nail dystrophy (canaliform dystrophy of Heller)

Diagnosis

Brittle nails and possible superimposed irritant nail disease.

R.A. Norman, J. Endo, *Clinical Cases in Geriatric Dermatology,* Clinical Cases in Dermatology, DOI 10.1007/978-1-4471-4135-8_32, © Springer-Verlag London 2013

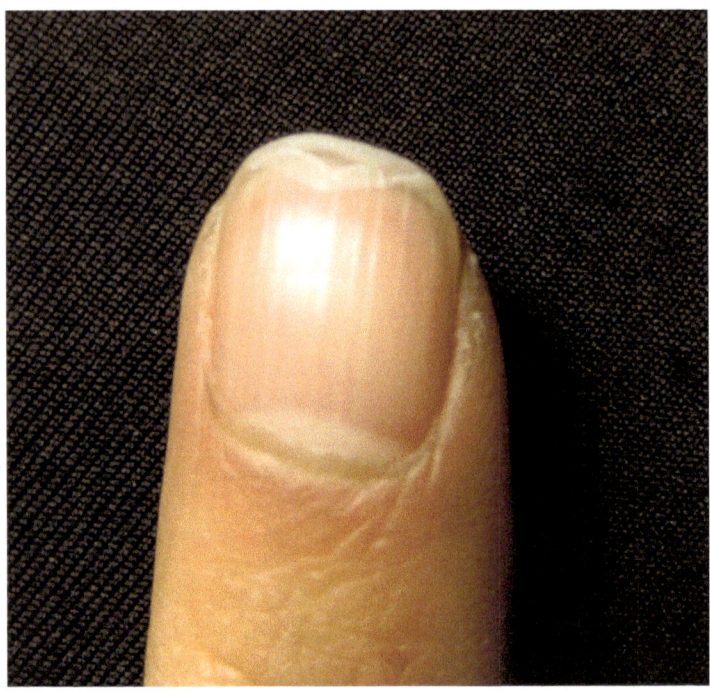

FIGURE 32.1 Patient complaining of thin, brittle nails that split very easily and have longitudinal ridges

Discussion

Brittle nails (peeling, raggedness, and/or ridging of the nail plate) are a common problem in the geriatric population, especially females (Sherber et al. 2011). In addition to normal senescence of nail production within the nail matrix, exogenous factors play a major role in pathophysiology. Repetitive hand washing or chemical irritants (e.g., nail cosmetics) degrade nail integrity. The result is nail splitting along the free edge. It is important to rule out other nutritional deficiencies that can also lead to brittle nail disease. Examples might include iron (classically presents as koilonychia or spoon nails), biotin, or cysteine deficiency (Hochman et al. 1993; Scher & Daniel 1997).

The mainstay of treatment is avoiding frequent hand washing with harsh detergents and avoiding manicures or nail cosmetics. A humectant such as ammonium lactate donates moisture to the nail plate and should be recommended after hand washing (Hochman et al. 1993). Limited data suggest biotin 2.5 mg daily supplementation, which is readily found at most pharmacies, health food stores, or grocery stores (Scheinfeld et al. 2007).

Differential Diagnoses

1. Onychomycosis is characterized by thickening and yellowing of the nails, as well as nail dystrophy (Hoy et al. 2012). Sometimes infected nails can crumble, but they do not typically split only on the distal nail plate (onychoschizia) as in this case.
2. Pterygium refers to abnormal adhesion of the nail plate to the surrounding nail apparatus. It can occur with fusion of the nail bed to the underside of the nail plate (ventral) or fusion of the proximal nail fold to the nail plate (dorsal). Lichen planus can cause dorsal pterygium or excessive nail roughness (trachyonychia) but not solely onychoschizia (Bolognia et al. 2008).
3. Psoriatic nail changes consist of pitting, oil spots, onychausis (nail thinning and excessive scale under nail plate) or onycholysis (separation of the nail plate off the nail bed). It is not characterized by only onychoschizia, which is splitting within the nail plate itself (Bolognia et al. 2008). Often, though not always, there is either family history of other cutaneous signs of psoriatic skin involvement.
4. Median nail dystrophy is an idiopathic condition that leads to a longitudinal depression of the midline of the nail plate with radiating "fir tree" like horizontal depressions. Some speculate it might be due to trauma from repetitive nail picking (Hoy et al. 2012).

Key Points

- Brittle nails are a common problem of aging.
- Barring an underlying medical or nutritional cause of the brittle nails, patients are recommended to avoid nail cosmetic products, minimize repeated wet-dry exposures of the fingers, and use humectants.
- Oral biotin supplementation and topical retinoids have modest evidence as second-line therapy.

References

Bolognia J, Jorizzo JL, Rapini RP. Dermatology. St. Louis: Mosby/Elsevier; 2008.

Hochman LG, Scher RK, Meyerson MS. Brittle nails: response to daily biotin supplementation. Cutis. 1993;51:303–5. cutaneous medicine for the practitioner.

Hoy NY, Leung AK, Metelitsa AI, Adams S. New concepts in median nail dystrophy, onychomycosis, and hand, foot, and mouth disease nail pathology. ISRN Dermatol. 2012;2012: 680163.

Scheinfeld N, Dahdah MJ, Scher R. Vitamins and minerals: their role in nail health and disease. J Drugs Dermatol. 2007;6:782–7.

Scher RK, Daniel CR. Nails: therapy, diagnosis, surgery. Philadelphia: Saunders; 1997.

Sherber NS, Hoch AM, Coppola CA, Carter EL, Chang HL, Barsanti FR, et al. Efficacy and safety study of tazarotene cream 0.1 % for the treatment of brittle nail syndrome. Cutis. 2011;87:96–103. cutaneous medicine for the practitioner.

Erratum

Clinical Cases in Geriatric Dermatology

By Robert A. Norman and Justin Endo

ISBN 978-1-4471-4134-1

P 147, 2nd paragraph should read:

"The hair pull test is considered positive when **more** than four telogen hairs (clubbed roots) are removed with a gentle tug and is highly suggestive of telogen effluvium"

R.A. Norman, J. Endo, *Clinical Cases in Geriatric Dermatology,* Clinical Cases in Dermatology, DOI 10.1007/978-1-4471-4135-8_33, © Springer-Verlag London 2013

Index

R.A. Norman, J. Endo, *Clinical Cases in Geriatric
Dermatology,* Clinical Cases in Dermatology,
DOI 10.1007/978-1-4471-4135-8,
© Springer-Verlag London 2013